PROFESSOR GABRIEL KUNE M̲ ̲ ̲ ̲ (England) FRACS FACS is Professor of Surgery Emeritus, University of Melbourne. He has been in the forefront of cancer research and cancer surgery for 30 years, and has published widely on cancer control, with a major focus on the prevention and early detection of cancer. A past Hunterian Professor of the Royal College of Surgeons of England, he has lectured extensively in Australia, New Zealand, USA, UK, Europe, Japan and South America. Professor Kune is passionately committed to the future successful control of all human cancers.

Annegret Nippa / Peter Herbstreuth (ed.)
Along the Gulf
From Basra to Muscat – Photographs by Hermann Burchardt.

ISBN: 978-389930-070-3 / bilingual German-English

The book explores the Arabian Gulf around 1900 through the eyes of Hermann Burchardt, a man without a political mission and no economical interests, merely intended "to take up a picture". Hermann Burchardt ist the answer to various turn-of-the-century exoticisms, sobering people's fantasies about the Orient. He saw the truth of photography in a sequential alignment of various perspectives as opposed to the single image. His mirrorings aimed to create a tension as regards interpretation, appearing as curious as reality itself.

Ali Hassan Jama
Who cares about Somalia?
Hassan's Ordeal - Reflections on a Nation's Future

ISBN 978-3-89930-075-8

This book is about a Somali civil war and the fall of the Siad Barre regime. It is about how people living there at the time did really suffer from it as a result. Although it principally relates to a family, the book tells an applicable story of flight, provisional shelter and finally exile. It is also about the political history of Somalia and about Somali ethnicity in general; and the book discusses the future of the Nation and how international and regional powers are involved in playing their sometimes influential roles in its intricate and complicated political path. For Somalis, international observers, historians and scholars alike one hopes these few lines shall offer some ideas to ponder and some more food for thought.

www.schiler.de

REDUCING THE ODDS

A MANUAL FOR THE PREVENTION OF CANCER

GABRIEL KUNE MD

ALLEN & UNWIN

First published in 1999
Allen & Unwin
9 Atchison Street, St Leonards NSW 1590 Australia
Phone: (61 2) 8425 0100
Fax: (61 2) 9906 2218
E-mail: frontdesk@allen-unwin.com.au
Web: http://www.allen-unwin.com.au

National Library of Australia
Cataloguing-in-Publication entry:

Kune, Gabriel A.
   Reducing the odds: a manual for the prevention of cancer.

   Bibliography.
   Includes index.
   ISBN 1 86508 028 4.

   1. Cancer—Prevention—Popular works. 2. Cancer—
   Etiology—Popular works. I. Title.

616.994052

Set in 11/13 pt Bembo by DOCUPRO, Sydney
Printed by Griffin Press Pty Ltd, Adelaide

10 9 8 7 6 5 4 3 2 1

Dedicated to pioneers of the science of prevention
and early detection of human cancer
Dr Denis Burkitt, Sir Richard Doll, Dr George Papanicolaou,
Dr Sidney Winawer, Dr Ernst Wynder

Contents

PART II   THE VARIOUS CAUSES OF CANCER • PREVENTIVE ACTION TO TAKE

Foreword

To prevent cancer effectively, it is necessary to have an understanding of what causes this disease. Toward this end, scientists have carried out a great number of studies over the past 20 years aimed at finding the causes of cancer. This research has been complicated by the fact that cancer is neither a single nor simple disease. Cancer is actually a complex group of diseases that result partly from genetic changes affecting cell growth and partly from influences on cell growth that are related to lifestyle choices and to various factors found in the physical surroundings of the workplace, home and other environments. A great deal of information, collected across many studies, suggests that the risk for a majority of human cancers can be reduced by primary prevention approaches, that is, by making changes in certain lifestyle habits, such as diet and smoking. To illustrate, vegetables, fruits, whole grains, dietary fibre, and perhaps certain vitamins and minerals appear to protect against cancer, whereas dietary fat, excessive calories, obesity, and alcohol seem to increase cancer risk. Some cancers can be prevented by eliminating exposures to specific environmental carcinogens, such as asbestos. Even if an inherited tendency for cancer is present, primary prevention measures may reduce cancer risk in some cases. Also, individuals with inherited tendencies will benefit from early detection of either precancerous conditions or very small tumours before they cause symptoms—which have the best chance of being cured by early treatment—by using special testing procedures.

This book, by Gabriel Kune, MD, is a readable, highly practical and current guide to cancer prevention. The guide emphasises that individuals, whether they are at average risk or high risk for developing cancer, can take action that may reduce their risk.

It provides a brief explanation of how cancer develops, explains the difference between primary and secondary prevention clearly, and provides basic information about the more common types of cancer. It discusses, in appropriate detail, major factors that can influence cancer risk, including genetic susceptibility, lifestyle choices—specifically, diet, tobacco use, alcohol use, sun exposure, physical activity, sexual activity and stress—and certain carcinogens that may be found in either the workplace or the home. Also, it describes the tests that are commonly used to screen for various types of cancer and outlines the current recommendations for using these tests.

The significant worth of a well thought out approach to prevention and early detection in reducing the chances of developing cancer needs to be more widely recognised by the general population. All too often, individuals do not have the knowledge required to carry out a realistic evaluation of their own cancer risk, which is an important first step in devising an effective cancer prevention approach.

Perhaps one of the most valuable aspects of this book is the systematic way in which it explains how the reader can use the information presented, in collaboration with a medical practitioner, to assess his or her personal cancer risk level and to develop a personal cancer prevention programme.

DR PETER GREENWALD, MD
Director
Division of Cancer Prevention
National Cancer Institute
Bethesda, Maryland, USA

Introduction

> *Most of us at some time during our adult life fear that we will develop a cancer. In fact, we have about one chance in three of developing a serious cancer during our lifetime. This risk can be halved for most people, and this book describes how it can be done.*

Cancer remains an important cause of early death in most communities of the world. Unfortunately, it often appears at a productive and successful stage of our lives, causing much fear, anxiety, sadness and despair. It has been known for centuries that the prevention of any illness is much better and much cheaper than its cure. Simple and very effective ways to prevent many illnesses are at our disposal, yet many of us continue with unhealthy life habits, and so we fail to avoid various illnesses, including cancer. In the 1996 September issue of the *Scientific American*, the current position of cancer prevention was stated very clearly.

Most types of cancer are to a large extent preventable with today's knowledge and technologies. The "war on cancer", primarily fought by searching for improved cancer treatments, has met with limited success and should be better balanced by more extensive efforts in prevention.

WHAT THIS BOOK IS ABOUT

This book deals exclusively with the prevention and early detection of cancers; it is comprehensive and provides the most current information, explained in simple, non-technical terms.

This book provides two distinct strategies, the first of which is cancer prevention. The book presents the causes of various cancers, and describes what we can do to avoid these cancers altogether, or at least to diminish our chances of developing a cancer. This is called *primary prevention of cancer*, and it will become our main weapon in the future against the cancer epidemic of the world.

The second strategy, distinct from primary prevention of cancer, is the *early detection of cancer using screening tests*. Most small cancers can be cured if found early and preferably before they cause symptoms. The early detection of such symptomless cancers and precancerous conditions, usually by the use of special tests, is an important part of this book. It has been predicted that early detection using existing forms of treatment is likely to save many lives in the future. You will find that this process is sometimes also referred to as *secondary prevention of cancer*, especially if it involves the removal of precancerous conditions, such as bowel polyps or skin moles.

The book is divided into four parts. The first is a brief explanation of how cancer develops, followed by a short description of the basic principles of cancer prevention. The several causes of different cancers are then summarised to provide an overview of the risk of cancer in an individual.

In the second part of the book, each cancer cause is discussed separately in detail, covering inherited causes, the role of dietary factors in cancer causation, tobacco use, alcohol consumption, excessive sunlight, physical inactivity, sexual practices and life stresses, as well as cancer-producing agents in the home, in the environment and in the workplace. Within each chapter of a particular cancer cause, such as smoking or diet, precise and clear recommendations are made for effective preventive action.

The third part describes the primary prevention and the early detection of individual cancers in detail, covering cancers of the colon and rectum, breast, lung, cervix, uterus, ovary, stomach, prostate, malignant melanoma and other skin cancers, and briefly also several other cancers which are less commonly encountered, namely cancers of the anus, bladder, brain, gallbladder, kidney, liver, mouth and throat, oesophagus, pancreas, penis, sarcomas, testicle, thyroid, vagina and vulva as well as leukaemias and lymphomas.

The fourth and final part of the book is a comprehensive cancer prevention programme which can be tailored to every individual's particular background and needs. This is followed by a glossary of technical terms explained simply, references for further reading, and addresses of cancer organisations.

So this book is first best read in its entirety, and then the reader can come back to it, and use it as a practical manual for the effective prevention and early detection of cancer.

WHO THIS BOOK IS WRITTEN FOR

Concern or fear that a cancer may develop

Those who for some reason fear that they will develop a cancer in the future and wish to improve their chances will find this book of particular interest. If you are one of the concerned individuals, you will find that your fears can often be allayed. On the other hand, if you are really at risk for cancer, you can take positive and effective steps to lower your risk, or at least have the likelihood that a cancer or a precancerous condition will be detected at a curable stage. You may also be able to help a family member or a friend who is reluctant to find out personally about cancer risk and cancer prevention.

Relative with cancer

You may be someone who has one or more relatives who have had a cancer. There may be a fear that you or other members of the family will also develop a cancer because of inheritance. This would be an excellent reason for reading this book.

Cancer has been successfully treated in the past

This is not a book about the treatment of various cancers. Several popular books have already been written on cancer treatment. If you or a member of your family or a friend have had a cancer treated in the past, you will find that this book does not provide any details on symptoms, means of diagnosis, treatment, or your chances of survival or cure following treatment. However, you will find out whether you are at risk of having another cancer in the future, and if so, what you can do about its prevention or early detection.

'Nothing is terrible except fear itself' wrote Francis Bacon in 1623. Many scientists have concluded, as did Francis Bacon over 350 years ago, that the fear of a cancer developing can be worse than the cancer itself. However, if informed, you can overcome this fear, and most importantly, you can take positive steps to avoid cancer.

Health professionals

This book is written in the first instance for a general readership. However, medical practitioners, nurses, pharmacists, public health workers, counsellors in cancer support groups, health policy makers and other health professionals, who regularly advise the community on various aspects of health promotion and illness prevention would also find the up-to-date and comprehensive information provided in this book useful in their professional practice.

> *This book will allay fears and concerns about the development of cancer, and will point the way to a happy and enjoyable style of living, in which the chances of developing cancer can be halved, or should a cancer develop, the likelihood of its early discovery increased so that a likely cure by currently available treatment may be achieved.*

PART I

WHAT IS CANCER?
WHAT IS CANCER PREVENTION?
WHO IS AT RISK FOR CANCER?

1

What is cancer? Why and how cancer develops

This brief explanation of what a cancer is and why and how it develops, will help in the understanding of how prevention and early detection of various cancers can be achieved.

WHAT IS CANCER?

The human body consists of about 3 trillion cells, the body's tiny building blocks seen only under a microscope. In the middle of each cell is a structure, the *nucleus*, which is full of *deoxyribonucleic acid* (DNA), and contains about 100,000 *genes* which control every activity of the cell. Damage to DNA, for example by tobacco or other harmful substances, can lead to a normal cell becoming cancerous. The cells are bound together by connective tissue to form a variety of organs, such as the skin, heart, lung or liver, together making up the body. Each tissue and organ has cells which have their individual shapes, structures and functions to fulfil. Every cell has a regular lifespan in every organ; it then dies and is replaced by the division of young cells. The body controls the death of old cells and the birth of new cells.

3

A malignant tumour, or cancer, usually develops from a single cell which undergoes uncontrolled division and growth. It escapes from the normal restraints on growth and division, and in a way becomes 'immortal'. If this uncontrolled division of cells remains unchecked, the cancer enlarges, becomes a visible or a palpable lump and causes symptoms. The cancer cells can then invade the surrounding normal tissues. Cancer cells can also travel to distant parts of the body through the lymphatic system or through the circulation, such as from the large bowel to the liver, lung or brain. Such a distant tumour is called a *metastasis*, or a *metastatic cancer*. Figure 1 is a simplified drawing of a skin cancer, a malignant melanoma, developing from a normal skin cell. It shows invasion of the surrounding tissues and also distant spread to lymph nodes and other organs.

A malignant tumour can develop in any part of the body. There are over 100 different types of malignant tumours. There is no part of the body which is immune from cancer, the common sites being the skin, lung, breast, colon and rectum, prostate, cervix, uterus, ovary, stomach and pancreas. The commonest cancer cell type is called *carcinoma* (skin, lung, breast, colon, rectum, prostate, cervix, uterus, ovary, stomach, gullet, pancreas), and these, with the much rarer *sarcoma* (bone, muscle, cartilage, fat, blood vessel, connective tissue) are called *solid tumours*. If the cells normally move or float in liquid, they are called *fluid tumours*, such as cancers of the blood cells, *leukaemias*.

WHY AND HOW CANCER DEVELOPS

Almost every moment of our life our body encounters substances or agents which get to various parts of the body and which can damage young cells at their most vulnerable stage, that is, when they are dividing. The important cancer agents include smoking, certain aspects of diet, alcohol, radiation, occupational carcinogens, and environmental pollutants. A small proportion of people inherit the propensity to develop a particular cancer, but in over 90%, the cancer develops because of

Figure 1: An example of the ways cancer spreads, here illustrated by the skin cancer, malignant melanoma

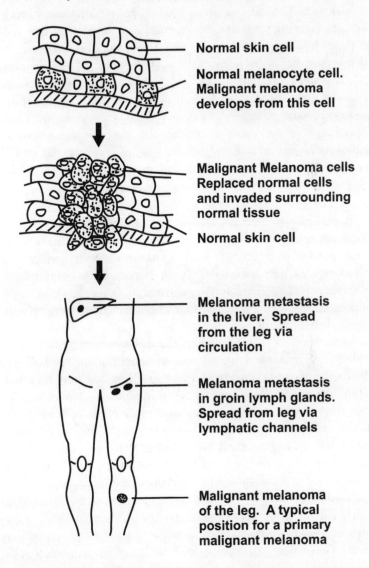

Normal skin cell

Normal melanocyte cell. Malignant melanoma develops from this cell

Malignant Melanoma cells Replaced normal cells and invaded surrounding normal tissue

Normal skin cell

Melanoma metastasis in the liver. Spread from the leg via circulation

Melanoma metastasis in groin lymph glands. Spread from leg via lymphatic channels

Malignant melanoma of the leg. A typical position for a primary malignant melanoma what we eat, drink, smoke or what is present in our work or home environment. The genetic coding, located on DNA in the cell nucleus and containing about 100 000 genes, determines every single characteristic, appearance, structure and function of that cell and therefore of the entire body. This allows the body to preserve and maintain its special identity. It is at the stage of cell division that the genetic material is most vulnerable to damage by certain substances such as tobacco, alcohol, ultraviolet rays, certain foods, asbestos fibre and others—all of these we may call *carcinogens*. Each of these agents can cause a genetic change or *mutation* in the dividing cell. The new cell produced in this way may be under less control than the normal cell, and may commence to divide and grow in an uncontrolled manner.

> *The change from a normal cell to a cancer cell is usually in several stages. Several insults by cancer-producing agents damage DNA, and this results in several cell mutations, which eventually produce a cancer cell.*

As a result of these genetic changes or mutations in the dividing cell, produced by various carcinogens, the normal cell will change its appearance in several steps. The first step is a rapid multiplication of cells, a process called *hyperplasia*. The next step is that the cell will become an abnormal or *dysplastic* cell, a process called *dysplasia*, in which the affected cells look different from a normal cell when examined under the microscope. This is not a cancer, but it is a first step in the development of a cancer. It can be called a *precancerous* or *premalignant* condition.

Another or alternative pathway of change or mutation as a result of damage by carcinogens, is from a normal cell into a *benign* or *innocent tumour*, such as an adenomatous polyp of the bowel. These benign tumours look different from normal cells when viewed under the microscope. These tumours are usually precancerous conditions just like the dysplastic cell, and they can change into an actual cancer.

As a result of further damage to either the abnormal or dysplastic cell, or to the benign tumour, the next step is that these precancerous cells change into an actual cancer when dividing. Initially these cancer cells do not have the ability to invade local tissues or to spread, and in some instances remain unchanged for months or even years. Such microscopic cancers are called *carcinoma-in-situ* or *in-situ cancer*. If there are only a few cancer cells, these can often be destroyed or their progress halted by the normal immune system of the body. However, if these few cancer cells are not destroyed, after any further DNA damage resulting in further mutations, the next stage is an uncontrolled multiplication of these cancer cells. These cells can then invade the local normal tissues—this is called an *invasive cancer*. With further growth the cancer becomes a visible or palpable swelling, a lump which can be seen or felt or recognised when examined on an x-ray or ultrasound examination. The final stage is when such a cancer not only invades the local normal tissue, but some of the cancer cells detach themselves, and travel either by the lymphatic channels into the lymph glands, or by the blood stream to other distant organs such as the liver, lung or brain. Such a distant tumour is called a *metastasis*. This represents an advanced and usually incurable stage. Figure 2 is a simplified diagram which illustrates the steps in the process just described of why and how a human cancer develops.

Cancer is a multistep process which develops over a long period of time, usually over several years, and sometimes over decades.

Figure 2: This diagram shows the causes of cancer, resulting in a series of genetic changes, with the eventual development of a cancer cell from a normal cell

Cancer causes

Tobacco, some foods, alcohol, excessive sunlight, occupational hazards (asbestos, radiation etc), environmental and household pollutants (radon gas, tobacco smoke etc) and others. Some people are born with an inherited propensity for cancer.

DNA damage and mutations

Cancer-producing agents cause repeated damage to DNA and result in a series of genetic changes or mutations. Mutations are already present in those with inherited propensity for cancer.

Change from normal cell to cancer cell

This occurs in several steps and usually over several years.

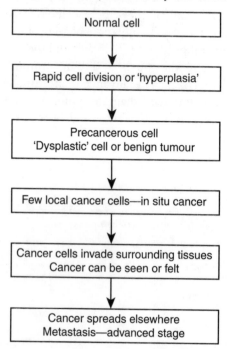

WHAT CAN BE DONE ABOUT CANCER?

We are subject to attack by many cancer-producing agents every day, and it is only occasionally that a person develops a cancer as a result. Fortunately, we also have many inbuilt ways of neutralising these cancer-producing agents. More precisely, we have inbuilt *cancer suppressing genes*, we have *genes that repair damaged DNA*, and we have our *immune system* that is able to destroy cancer cells or precancerous cells. If there are only a few cancer cells present in the body, part of the cellular immune system is mobilised, and one of our circulating white cells, *killer T cell*, can attack and destroy these cancer cells.

We can also take action ourselves, change our life habits and thereby diminish the risk of a cancer developing in our body. This is called *primary prevention*. Moreover, thanks to advances in modern medical science, even if a small cancer or a precancerous condition does develop in the body, we now have many ways of finding these and can remove them before they cause irreparable harm. This is called *early detection using screening tests*. This book focuses on both the primary prevention of cancer and on its early detection using screening tests.

2

What is cancer prevention?

*It is a wise man's part, rather to avoid
sickness, than to wishe for medicines.*

Sir Thomas More (1478–1535)

There are two ways in which cancer can be prevented. The
first is to discover the causes, and then remove or avoid these
causes. This is called *primary prevention*. Examples of primary
prevention are the avoidance of sunburn to prevent skin cancer,
quitting smoking to prevent lung cancer, and many others
suggested in this book. The second main avenue of prevention
is to *identify a precancerous condition* before it becomes a cancer,
usually by using special tests, and then to remove it, or to *identify
an early cancer* before it has spread and remove it at that time.
This is called *screening for cancer*, or *early detection using screening
tests* or, for precancerous conditions, *secondary prevention*. Examples of this are the removal of an early breast cancer, or the
removal of precancerous 'sunspots' on the skin, or the removal
of precancerous bowel polyps, and several others which will be
described throughout this book.

PRIMARY PREVENTION

> *The good doctor pays constant attention*
> *to keeping people well,*
> *so that there will be no sickness.*
>
> *Lin An (died about 120 BC)*

If the main cause or causes of a particular cancer are known, such as smoking in lung cancer, or excessive sunlight and sunburn in skin cancer, then avoiding these cancer-producing agents will decrease the chances of developing cancer.

With some cancers the causes are not well understood and therefore effective primary prevention advice specific to that cancer cannot be given. Effective primary prevention can be advised, for example, for cancers of the lung, skin, and large bowel, but there are as yet no well-established primary prevention measures for breast or prostate cancer. For those cancers in which the causes are not well known, we need to largely rely on screening tests for their early detection.

Some advantages of primary prevention

Primary preventive measures are almost always performed by the person involved, so you are in complete control of the situation. They are usually an inexpensive means of lowering the chances of developing a particular cancer, as they need little or no professional guidance. Excellent examples of this are avoidance or quitting smoking, changing one's diet, and avoiding excessive exposure to sunlight. Primary prevention should be harmless and without risk, practical, and should fit in with the broader practices of health promotion.

Some obstacles to primary prevention

Although primary prevention measures are usually simple and cheap, they can involve major changes in life habits, and herein lies one of the main problems associated with the primary prevention of cancer. We need to be both aware and motivated to make these changes. This can be difficult, particularly if some of these habits are addictive, such as smoking or excessive alcohol use, or when the habit is deeply entrenched, such as a particular type of diet. Moreover, young adults often feel they are invincible, and are not motivated to change some habits, especially if they are fashionable, well promoted, or perceived as giving pleasure or prestige. The great value and power of prevention is not fully appreciated by the community at large, partly because scientific advances in the treatment of cancer rather than its prevention receive the most publicity, and partly because human nature is such that it would prefer the 'magic bullet treatment', instead of adopting changes in established life habits. Although a lot is known about the primary prevention of several cancers, unhealthy cancer-producing habits persist with many of us. A lot still needs to be done through education in order to promote cancer prevention. Hopefully this book will go some way towards that goal.

Early detection of cancer using screening tests

If there are means of identifying and removing precancerous conditions, or if it is possible to identify and remove early cancers before they have spread, then the growth of an invasive and potentially fatal cancer can be prevented.

An example of early detection involving precancerous conditions is the systematic removal of precancerous skin lesions such as sunspots, or some types of dark moles, before a skin cancer or a malignant melanoma develops. Other examples are the removal of precancerous bowel polyps with the use of a

12

colonoscope, or the removal of precancerous conditions of the cervix with a relatively simple operation.

Early detection of cancer using screening tests is usually performed on people who are apparently well; that is, they feel well and have no symptoms or complaints. This almost always involves a medical examination, and usually it also involves special tests, such as testing the bowel motions for minute quantities of blood (faecal occult blood testing) in order to detect precancerous bowel polyps or early bowel cancers, breast examination and mammography to detect early breast cancer, or vaginal examination and a cervix smear test to detect pre-cancerous states of the cervix or an early cervix cancer. This means that the method used in the early detection of cancer with screening tests is usually expensive and often carries some risk, whereas primary prevention is usually inexpensive with few risks or complications involved. The issues of cost, cost–benefit and risks involved become critical when mass screening of an entire population is being considered, such as screening for breast cancer, colorectal cancer or prostate cancer. There is a major distinction between the mass screening of an entire population and the screening of an individual who is motivated to seek screening for a cancer from a medical practitioner. This book deals almost exclusively with the practice of screening for the early detection of cancer in an individual who seeks advice from a medical practitioner, within the context of the traditional doctor–patient relationship. The discussion of mass screening for cancer is largely outside the scope of this book.

There are also exciting prospects for improved ways of early diagnosis of cancer and of precancerous conditions which are currently being developed, using methods which have little risk to the individual. Some of these new tests involve genetic blood testing, others involve the identification of damaged DNA, and some involve the identification of enzyme markers in the body which signal the presence of an early cancer, or of a precan-cerous condition.

The early detection of cancer or of precancerous conditions is usually more complex than primary prevention. Also, early

Table 2.1: Comparison of primary prevention with early detection using screening tests

Form of prevention	What is done	How it is done	Positives	Problems
Primary prevention	*Avoid the cause* For example • Avoid sunburn • Avoid smoking *Reverse the cause* For example • Quit smoking • Change diet *Improve immunity* For example • Hepatitis vaccination	Guided self-help	Usually cheap Usually simple No risks involved Can prevent other illnesses also, such as heart disease	May involve major changes in behaviour and daily living There can be a problem associated with breaking established and/or addictive habits
Early detection using screening tests for cancer	*Remove precancerous condition* For example • Sunspots, moles • Bowel polyps *Remove early curable cancer* For example • Early breast cancer • Early cervix cancer • Early colorectal cancer	Medical examination + special tests. For example • Mammography • Testing stool for blood • Cervix smear test	Does not usually require changes in life habits	Usually expensive Cost is usually a major issue in mass screening Some tests have risks and complications Major issue in mass screening Screening may miss precancerous conditions or early cancer (false negative test) Screening may falsely suggest cancer is present (false positive test) requiring unnecessary tests, and potential for complications or distress

detection often involves an invasion of the body because of the special tests which need to be done, and this is much more expensive than primary prevention. These two methods of prevention are compared and summarised in Table 2.1. This table clearly suggests that primary prevention is preferable to early detection using screening tests, provided primary prevention is possible.

CAN ALL CANCERS BE PREVENTED OR DETECTED EARLY?

Unfortunately not all cancers can be prevented or identified early, and at a stage when they can be cured. In an ideal world, which is free from all outside cancer-producing agents, three cancers out of four can probably be prevented or at least detected early and cured. About one in four cancers cannot be prevented even under ideal circumstances, partly because the body can itself produce agents which damage DNA, partly because there can be genetic accidents during cell division which are not repaired, and partly because we don't know everything about cancer causation and early detection.

> *A realistic estimate for developed countries is that about half of all cancers are preventable, or at least detectable at an early and curable stage.*

3

Who is at risk for cancer?

In developed countries a large proportion of the adult population is at risk of developing some type of a cancer during their lifetime. This is because the majority of us who live in a so-called Western or developed country, have a lifestyle and live in an environment which for various reasons puts us at risk for cancer. Some of us also have an inherited predisposition to cancer. This chapter provides a bird's-eye view of the several reasons why a person may have an increased cancer risk.

> *Most of us would be considered as average risk for cancer, and not low risk, because the usual Western lifestyle and environment in itself poses cancer risks. Reading this book further you'll discover that if you are in the average risk category, you can put yourself into the low risk group for cancer by changing your life habits and by changing your home and work environment.*

In Western communities there is a small group of individuals who are indeed at low risk for cancer, and usually they have placed themselves in this fortunate position by their own actions.

These are individuals who eat an exceptionally healthy diet (lots of vegetables, fruit, cereals, starchy foods, fibre, fish and little fat and meat and not excessive calories), are not overweight, do not smoke, do not drink alcohol excessively, perform physical activity regularly, avoid excessive sunshine, and avoid stress, or deal with stress using special techniques such as relaxation or meditation. If at the same time they have no family history of any type of cancer, nor any suggestion of an inherited predisposition to cancer, they would be at a very low risk indeed for cancer.

At the other end of the scale are individuals at an elevated risk of developing cancer during their lifetime because of particular characteristics in their family, because of certain factors in their past medical health, because of certain life habits such as eating an unhealthy diet, smoking, drinking excessively, being physically inactive and leading a very stressful life, or because they are in an environment at work, at home or in the neighbourhood in which there are cancer-producing substances present. Individuals who belong to one or more of these groups are designated as being at an increased risk for cancer.

PEOPLE AT INCREASED RISK FOR CANCER

There are several reasons why an individual may be at higher than average risk for developing a particular cancer. I must stress that there is no certainty that in fact cancer will develop, simply the chances are increased compared to someone who is at average risk. For example, an average risk individual in a developed country has about a 1 in 20 chance of developing bowel cancer (cancer of the colon or rectum), but if they are at high risk, say because of a strong family history of bowel cancer or because of unusual life habits such as a combination of a poor diet, high smoking level and a high alcohol intake, then the chances of developing bowel cancer during their lifetime might increase to 1 in 10, or even 1 in 5.

Inherited cancers

Those who have an inherited predisposition to cancer fall into two groups, namely a tiny group who are at a very high risk of developing a particular cancer, and a much larger group who are only at a somewhat higher than average risk. Fortunately, those with an inherited risk can now usually be identified early, so that their potential cancer can be prevented, or if not prevented, at least found early and at a stage when it is still curable. The inherited aspects of cancer are discussed further in Chapter 4.

Inherited high cancer risk

There is a small group of individuals who are at a high risk (say 1 chance in 2) of developing a certain cancer because of a very strong inherited tendency. Although such families are uncommon, it is important to identify members of these families. A lot can now be done either to prevent these cancers occurring, or to identify early cancers and remove them at a stage when they can be cured permanently. Table 3.1 lists the conditions which give rise to a high cancer risk in a family.

Inherited above average cancer risk

Another and somewhat larger group than the families just described, are individuals who have a higher than average risk for certain cancers, because a family member has a particular cancer, or because of some inherited personal characteristic such as fair skin, which with excessive sun exposure, predisposes an individual to skin cancer. Table 3.2 describes those who are at a higher than average risk of developing certain cancers because of an inherited predisposition.

Certain past illnesses and medical treatment

Some past medical conditions, and several forms of medical or surgical treatment received in the past, are associated with an increased level of risk for certain cancers. The important medical

18

Table 3.1: Inherited conditions which indicate a high cancer risk

Name of condition	Site of cancer
Familial adenomatous polyposis (FAP)	Colon or rectal cancer mainly *also* Cancer of the stomach, duodenum and small bowel
Hereditary non-polyposis colorectal cancer (HNPCC), sometimes referred to as Lynch syndrome	Colon or rectal cancer mainly *also* Uterine and ovarian cancer, gastric cancer, pancreatic and biliary cancer, urinary system cancer
Breast-ovarian cancer syndrome (BOCS)	Breast cancer Ovarian cancer
Xeroderma pigmentosum	Malignant melanoma Non-melanoma skin cancer
Familial dysplastic naevus syndrome (DNS), also called familial atypical multiple mole melanoma (FAMMM)	Malignant melanoma

Table 3.2: Inherited characteristics which suggest higher than average cancer risk

Recognition of inherited characteristic	Site of cancer
History of the following cancers in near relative (parents, brothers, sisters, children, grandparents, uncles and aunts): Colon or rectal cancer Colon or rectal adenomatous polyps Breast cancer Prostate cancer Lung cancer Ovarian cancer Gastric cancer Pancreas cancer Liver cancer	Same site as in family member
Type A blood	Stomach
Fair hair (blonde or red), fair complexion, blue eyes, freckles, skin burns easily with sun exposure	Melanoma Non-melanoma skin cancer

Table 3.3: Medical conditions which increase cancer risk

Medical condition	Site of cancer
Previously removed cancer or benign tumour, such as adenoma or papilloma of:	
Colon or rectum	Remaining colon or rectum
Breast	Remaining breast or other breast
Ovary	Remaining ovary or other ovary
Skin	Other parts of skin
Lung	Remaining lung or other lung
Previously removed cancer of colon or rectum, or breast, or ovary, or uterus	Cancer in any one of the other organs listed
Lymphoma or leukaemia (and chemotherapy treatment)	Skin cancer
Abnormal (dysplastic) cells on biopsy of:	
Breast	Breast cancer
Colon or rectum	Colon or rectal cancer
Cervix	Cervix cancer
Uterus	Uterine cancer
Gullet (oesophagus)	Gullet (oesophagus) cancer
Stomach	Stomach (gastric) cancer
Skin	Skin cancer
Chronic lung disease, such as chronic bronchitis, emphysema, scarred lungs	Lung cancer
Ulcerative colitis Crohn's disease	Colon or rectal cancer
Genital herpes, genital warts or anal warts	Cervix cancer, penis cancer, anal cancer
Hepatitis B carrier Hepatitis C	Liver cancer
Human immunodeficiency virus (HIV), which progresses to acquired immunodeficiency syndrome (AIDS)	Lymphoma, Kaposi sarcoma
Heartburn over many years	Gullet (oesophagus) cancer
Pernicious anaemia	Stomach (gastric) cancer
Diabetes	Pancreas cancer, uterine cancer, ovarian cancer
Chronic pancreatitis	Pancreas cancer

conditions and forms of treatment which may lead to cancers at certain sites are described in Table 3.3.

Table 3.4 lists the various forms of medical, surgical or radiation treatment which predispose an individual to cancer in various parts of the body.

Table 3.4: Previous medical or surgical treatment and elevated cancer risk

Previous treatment	Site of cancer
Radiation to chest	Breast cancer, lung cancer
Radiation to neck	Thyroid cancer
Radiation to pelvis	Sigmoid colon cancer, rectal cancer, ovarian cancer, uterine cancer, bladder cancer
Radiation to skin	Skin cancer
Hormone replacement therapy containing only oestrogens	Breast cancer, uterine cancer, ovarian cancer
Partial removal of stomach (partial gastrectomy) for non-malignant condition	Stomach (gastric) cancer
Kidney transplant Chemotherapy to treat malignant tumours	Skin cancer

Certain life habits

There are several daily activities and habits in Western communities which predispose individuals to various cancers. The most important of these habits are an unhealthy diet and smoking and, to a lesser extent, excessive alcohol consumption, physical inactivity, and possibly a stressful life and a poor capacity to cope with stress.

Diet

The type of diet which appears to be connected with cancer at several sites in the body is one in which there is a particularly low consumption of vegetables, fruit, cereals and starchy foods and therefore a low intake of total dietary fibre, and probably also a low consumption of fish. The other characteristics of this

Table 3.5: Diet-related cancers

Diet a proven cause	Diet a likely contributory cause
Colon cancer	Breast cancer
Rectal cancer	Prostate cancer
Adenomatous polyps of colon and rectum (precancerous tumours)	Stomach (gastric) cancer
	Gullet (oesophagus) cancer
	Pancreas cancer
	Uterine cancer
	Ovarian cancer
	Lung cancer
	Cervix cancer

diet are a high consumption of energy-rich foods, such as sugar and fat, as well as a high consumption of animal fat and meat. This type of diet is a cancer risk if followed over many years.

The opposite type of diet, with a particularly high consumption of vegetables, fruit, cereals, starch and total dietary fibre, a high consumption of fish, and a low consumption of energy-rich foods, as well as a low consumption of animal fat and meat, lowers your cancer risk and provides a degree of protection against various cancers. The dietary aspects of cancer, as well as the dietary prevention of various cancers, are discussed in detail in Chapter 5. Table 3.5 lists the cancers which appear to be related to dietary habits.

Tobacco

Smoking or tobacco use is an important cause of death and a particularly important cause of cancer death. It has been estimated that smoking is responsible for every third cancer death, and that 1 of 2 regular smokers will die prematurely from a smoking-related cancer. The relationship between smoking and tobacco use and the prevention of various smoking-related cancers is described in Chapter 6. Table 3.6 is a summary of smoking-related cancers.

Alcohol consumption

Excessive alcohol consumption is also an important contributory cause of cancer. The relationship between alcohol

Table 3.6: Smoking-related cancers

Smoking a proven cause	Smoking a likely contributory cause	Smoking a possible contributory cause
Lung cancer	Stomach (gastric) cancer	Colon cancer
Mouth cancer	Kidney cancer	Rectal cancer
Throat cancer	Cervix cancer	Primary liver cancer
Gullet (oesophagus) cancer	Colon adenomas (polyps)	Prostate cancer
Bladder cancer	Rectal adenomas (polyps)	Penis cancer
Pancreas cancer	Anal cancer	

Table 3.7: Alcohol-related cancers

Alcohol a proven cause	Alcohol a likely contributory cause
Mouth cancer	Colon cancer
Throat cancer	Rectal cancer
Gullet (oseophagus) cancer	Colon adenomas (polyps)
Primary liver cancer	Rectal adenomas (polyps)
	Breast cancer

consumption and the development of cancer is described in detail in Chapter 7. Table 3.7 indicates the cancer sites linked to excessive alcohol consumption.

Excessive sun exposure

Excessive exposure to sunlight, and particularly if this results in sunburn, and especially in those who are fair skinned and susceptible to sunburn, may lead to both non-melanoma skin cancer and to malignant melanoma (Chapter 8). Table 3.8 lists the cancers related to excessive sun exposure.

Table 3.8: Sun-related cancers

Malignant melanoma
Non-melanoma skin cancer
• basal cell carcinoma
• squamous cell carcinoma

Table 3.9: Physical inactivity and cancer risk sites

Colon cancer
Colon adenoma (polyp)
Breast cancer
Testicular cancer
Ovarian cancer
Prostate cancer
Uterine cancer

Physical inactivity

Leading an inactive or largely sedentary life and not participating in occupational or recreational physical activity regularly, has been shown to be a likely contributory cause, albeit small, of colon cancer and also of the main precancerous condition of colon cancer, a colonic adenomatous polyp.

Physical inactivity may also be a risk for some other cancers, and in particular cancers of the breast, uterus, ovary, prostate and testicle. However, the scientific evidence for these is less strong than that for colon tumours. The role of physical activity in cancer prevention is described in more detail in Chapter 9. Table 3.9 lists the parts of the body in which cancer risk rises because of an inactive life.

Sexual activity

Sexually transmitted diseases (STD), usually viruses, predispose an individual to certain cancers including cancers of the cervix, penis, anus, liver, as well as to lymphoma and sarcoma, as indicated in Table 3.10, and discussed in detail in Chapter 10.

Stressful life

Major life stresses as well as major losses in life, such as the loss of one's spouse or parent, or the loss of a job, take their toll on our health. In some individuals such a loss can be a trigger for the appearance and growth of a cancer, a cancer which up to that time had remained dormant. The relationship between stress and cancer prior to the onset of these stressful events, and what can be done about this, is described in Chapter 11.

Table 3.10: Sexually transmitted viruses predisposing to cancer

Virus involved	Type of cancer
Human papilloma virus (HPV) Herpes simplex II (genital herpes)	Cervix cancer Vaginal cancer Penis cancer Anal cancer
Human immunodeficiency virus (HIV), progresses to acquired immunodeficiency syndrome (AIDS)	Lymphoma Kaposi sarcoma
Hepatitis B virus Hepatitis C virus (uncommonly STD)	Liver cancer

Environmental effects

Cancer-producing substances can be present at work—asbestos fibre, pesticides, benzene, and many other chemicals and noxious substances. Exposure to these substances is dealt with in detail in Chapter 12. Cancer-producing agents also exist in the home or in the neighbourhood—passive inhalation of tobacco smoke, the use of pesticides, household cleaners and solvents, radon gas in houses, and exposure to low frequency electromagnetic fields in the neighbourhood. The possible role of these agents in the development of cancers is discussed in detail in Chapter 13. Although work, home and neighbourhood cancer effects do occur, they are responsible for cancers much less frequently than those caused by personal life habits, past illnesses, past treatment, or those due to an inherited tendency for cancer.

ESTIMATING PERSONAL CANCER RISK

You have by now an overview of how one begins to assess in a simple common-sense manner, whether a person has a higher than average chance of developing cancer. Simply by finding out about a history of cancer in the family, by recalling some specific illnesses and medical or surgical treatments which are listed in the previous tables in this chapter, by examining life habits in relation to diet, smoking, alcohol, exposure to sunlight, physical activity, life stresses, and then by examining the type of work that is done, as well as anything one may be exposed to at home or in the neighbourhood which may be cancer-producing, a very approximate assessment of personal cancer risk can be made.

The next few chapters of this book deal with individual aspects of cancer prevention, such as the inherited aspects of cancer, diet, smoking, alcohol consumption, exposure to sunlight, physical activity, exposure to cancer-producing agents at work, in the home and in the neighbourhood, as well as the role of the mind and stress in the development of cancer. In each of these chapters, the means for prevention will be described and precise recommendations will be made. Individual chapters will then be devoted to the prevention and early detection of particular cancers, namely cancers of the colon and rectum, breast, lung, prostate, skin, cervix, uterus, ovary, stomach, as well as several other less common cancers. An assessment of personal cancer risk and a personal programme for the prevention and early detection of cancers, which is to be used in collaboration with a medical practitioner, is then mapped out in the final chapter.

PART II

THE VARIOUS CAUSES OF CANCER
PREVENTIVE ACTION TO TAKE

4

Inherited cancer

*When an expert in genetics with a sense of humour
was asked whether insanity is inherited, she replied,
'Yes it is. You get it from your children!'*

*It is important to realise that at least nine of ten human
cancers are due to non-inherited causes. A tendency inherited
from our parents to develop cancer is fortunately not
common. In some families, however, cancer is inherited in
a regular manner just as eye colour or physical appearance
is inherited, and such families usually belong to what is
called* Inherited Family Cancer Syndromes. *More commonly, an inherited tendency for cancer is suspected simply
because other members of the family have been found to
have a cancer.*

In some families, bowel cancer is common or breast cancer is
common, and this is the important clue that there may be an
inherited basis for that cancer. In such situations, other members
of the family who have not been identified to have a cancer
are at a higher risk for that cancer than would otherwise be

expected. Those who inherit fair skin which burns easily with sun exposure are prone to skin cancer, if they have received excessive irradiation from the sun. In this category also are individuals who metabolise certain compounds too fast by chemical processes termed oxidation and acetylation, and because of this inherited characteristic are prone to colon and rectal cancer, if they also eat excessive amounts of heavily fried or heavily grilled meat. These last two examples reveal the interaction that may be present between inherited characteristics and lifestyle habits, which, when combined, can result in a cancer.

HOW CANCER IS INHERITED

One of the most important advances in the understanding of how a cancer develops has been the discovery that cancer has a genetic basis, as has already been described in Chapter 1. To explain this simply, imagine that every cell of the body contains a part called the *nucleus* which has in it a set of *chromosomes,* and that within each chromosome there are numerous *genes*. These genes control the appearance and function of every cell, and for that matter, of the whole body. When a cell divides, in order to replace cells which have died, the genes also divide and do so in such a way that two cells result. Each of these cells is a precise copy of the parent cell. In this way the chromosomes and genes are maintained and remain identical to the parent cell, retaining their normal appearance and function.

The genes which are associated with cancer development are present in the chromosomes normally, but they do not cause cancer unless they are faulty or damaged. Irrespective of whether they are inherited or develop during life as a consequence of cancer–producing substances, these faulty genes are referred to as *mutated genes*, or *mutations*. There some genes which protect the body from the development of a cancer, called *tumour suppressor genes*. Moreover, there are also genes, which could be termed *cancer-producing genes*, called *oncogenes*. In a small proportion of individuals, genes which are already mutated are inherited. More commonly, mutated genes are not inherited, but are the result of certain cancer-producing substances, such as those found in tobacco, some foods, or alcohol. These substances can damage the cell's DNA and change a normal gene into a cancer-producing gene while the cell is dividing. The change from a normal cell to a cancer cell usually does not occur in one step, and several mutations occur before an actual cancer cell develops from a normal cell.

INHERITED FAMILY CANCER SYNDROMES

Inherited family cancer syndromes are uncommon and only touch a few families. However, should such a syndrome be identified in a family, it is most important that each family member is aware of it, so that the right steps are taken to identify at an early and curable stage any cancer which may develop. Genetic counselling is now available in many centres for members of such families.

Inherited family cancers appear to be associated with one or more gene abnormalities, or mutations, which are inherited and which eventually lead to a particular and specific type of cancer. Because these gene abnormalities are present in all cells of the body, in some situations it is now possible to perform blood tests and detect those members of the family who are carrying the cancer-producing genes. These blood tests have been an enormous advance in the process of screening and counselling these families.

Since it is now commonplace to read or hear about some of these inherited mutated genes, their technical names and in brackets the cancer they are usually associated with are listed here: APC (familial adenomatous polyposis, colorectal cancer), MSH2, MLH1, PMS1, PMS2 (hereditary non-polyposis colorectal cancer), BRCA1 (breast and ovary cancer), BRCA2 (breast cancer), CDKN2 (melanoma, pancreas cancer), CDK4 (skin cancer), WT1, VHL (kidney cancer), NF1 (brain, nervous system cancer), *ret* (thyroid cancer).

Identification of family cancer syndromes

There are certain characteristics of the cancer in inherited family cancer syndromes. The five main cancer characteristics are:

- The cancer develops one or two decades earlier than in those whose cancer is of the non-inherited type.
- Several family members are affected by the same type of cancer, for example, colon cancer or breast cancer.
- The same type of cancer develops in several and usually successive generations of the family.
- Sometimes more than one type of cancer develops in a family, such as colon cancer, rectal cancer, breast cancer, uterine cancer.
- One or several specific chromosomal abnormalities are present in the affected family members.

It is some or all of these characteristics of the cancers in the family which would alert a family member or a medical practitioner to make a careful study of the family history, to draw a family tree and then to have genetic counselling which may include blood testing, provided that a blood test is available to detect the abnormal chromosomes.

Since not all members of the family will inherit the predisposition to a particular type of cancer, the blood tests are of immense value for two reasons:

- The family members who are shown to have the abnormal gene need to know that screening and regular follow-up and treatment is essential for them in order to detect and remove any precancerous condition or early cancer, so that they will have a normal lifespan.
- The family members who have definitely not inherited the cancer-producing gene can be reassured that they are at no

greater risk of developing that particular cancer than the rest of the population. This knowledge would help relieve unaffected family members of the psychological burden which is often present.

The best understood inherited family cancer syndromes are familial adenomatous polyposis (FAP) and hereditary non-polyposis colorectal cancer (HNPCC), and these will be described first.

Familial adenomatous polyposis (FAP)

In 100 consecutive individuals who are diagnosed as having large bowel cancer (colon or rectal cancer) only one will have the inherited condition of familial adenomatous polyposis (FAP). These individuals develop hundreds or sometimes thousands of adenomatous polyps in their large bowel, usually in their late teens, and if these innocent polyps remain untreated, invariably one or more cancers will later develop in these bowel polyps.

The condition is transmitted from one parent carrying an abnormal chromosome, so that about half the children of such a parent will develop polyposis. These bowel polyps appear because of an inherited abnormal gene on chromosome 5, called the *adenomatous polyposis coli gene* (APC). The treatment of this condition is by secondary prevention, which in this case means the surgical removal of the bowel containing the polyps at a time before a cancer of the colon or rectum has had a chance to develop from one of the many hundred bowel polyps.

As only half the members of an FAP family develop polyps and then cancer if the polyps are untreated, it is important to identify those family members who carry the APC gene. This can now be done using special blood tests, which became available in the early 1990s, and were a major advance in the screening of family members. Using these methods no false positive tests have so far been identified. However, it has become clear that these early methods of testing will miss 1 in 4 (25%) of those who in fact possess the abnormal APC gene. Because of these false negative tests new methods of testing those who are at risk for FAP have been evolved. One of the most promising of these newer tests has been developed recently in the USA, and is called *mono allelic mutation analysis* (MAMA). In conjunction with other tests, MAMA is able to detect at least 19 of 20 (95%) of those who have familial adenomatous polyposis.

Members of FAP families are at present best treated in special centres which have a comprehensive range of experts, including genetic counsellors, access to a molecular genetic laboratory for FAP blood testing, surgeons, gastroenterologists and other experts who are familiar with the total care of this uncommon inherited family syndrome.

Hereditary non-polyposis colorectal cancer (HNPCC)

About 4% of individuals who develop colorectal cancer do so because of inherited gene abnormalities which predispose them to colon or rectal cancer. The characteristics of such families are that they develop large bowel cancer at a young age, often some 20 or more years earlier than is the norm (such as at the age of 35–40), that bowel cancer has been identified in two or more family members, that bowel cancer has been noted in two or three generations, that there are not hundreds of polyps in the bowel (as there are in FAP), and that the family also suffers from an unusually large number of other cancers, in particular uterine and ovarian cancer in women, as well as stomach, pancreas and kidney cancer and cancer at other sites in both sexes. In the past, these cancers have been called *Lynch syndrome I* when the cancer in a family is limited to the large bowel, and *Lynch syndrome II* when the cancer occurs in a family in the large bowel as well as at other sites in the body. They were so named because of the untiring efforts of Dr Henry Lynch, an American physician, who spearheaded the recognition of this condition.

HNPCC, just as FAP, is also transmitted to only half the children of an affected individual. In recent years several mutated genes, the *DNA mismatch repair genes*, named MSH2, MLH1, PMS1 and PMS2, have been identified, and appear to be responsible for the development of HNPCC. Blood tests for these mutated genes are now beginning to be performed in special laboratories. At present these tests are much more difficult and more costly than blood tests for FAP, since each HNPCC family appears to have their own mutation pattern involving one of several genes on different chromosomes, whereas in FAP it is one gene on chromosome 5. Another problem is that as with FAP families, false positive tests have not been so far identified, however, using the early methods of mutational analysis, 1 in 2 (50%) of those with HNPCC will be missed. To overcome this unacceptably high number of false negative tests, additional tests have been recently developed, including MAMA, as described for FAP, which together with other tests can identify most individuals who have HNPCC.

At present, HNPCC families are usually identified by obtaining a careful history of large bowel cancer and of other cancers in the family, also noting that they are present in several family members, that they occur at earlier ages than would be expected and that they have been present in several generations. Clearly, genetic testing will become the most important screening method for those at risk for HNPCC, once the tests are simpler to perform and more informative in relation to negative results.

Members of an HNPCC family are at present best treated at special centres which have a comprehensive range of experts including genetic counsellors, as well as access to molecular genetics laboratories for HNPCC blood testing, surgeons, gastroenterologists, gynaecologists and other medical experts who are familiar with the treatment and secondary prevention of this inherited syndrome.

Breast-ovarian cancer syndrome (BOCS)

This is an uncommon inherited condition in which the women of the family have a high chance, though not a certainty, of developing breast cancer, or breast and ovarian cancer, at a younger age than is normally the case. It is possible that this condition is linked to the inheritance of an abnormal gene, BRCA1. There may also be a second gene, BRCA2, which may also be inherited. There is some uncertainty at present in relation to the precise interpretation of positive BRCA1 and BRCA2 genes, the practical aspects of which are discussed in Chapter 15, which deals with cancer of the breast.

Familial dysplastic naevus syndrome (DNS) or familial atypical multiple mole melanoma syndrome (FAMMM)

This is an uncommon inherited condition representing about 1% of all malignant melanomas, in which family members are liable to develop malignant melanoma from one of the many moles which these individuals usually possess. Tumours elsewhere in the body are also more common in these families than would otherwise be expected. The inherited tendency for this condition is probably due to a mutation of a gene called CDKN2A. Molecular biology research is proceeding rapidly to establish genetic testing using a blood test that can identify affected family members.

INHERITED CANCER SUSPECTED

Having dealt with the known inherited family cancer syndromes, we are left with a group of individuals who are not members of such families, nevertheless they have inherited a tendency to develop cancer. The inherited cancer is usually in a particular part of the body, most commonly in the colon, rectum or breast. Skin cancer, including malignant melanoma, and probably also cancer of the prostate, lung, stomach, uterus and ovary can be inherited. This tendency for inherited cancer is suspected when one or more members of the family have been identified with a cancer at one of these sites.

Proneness to inherited cancer—how would one know?

It is sometimes difficult to be sure that an individual is prone to inherited cancer just from the family history, since certain life habits which can lead to various cancers are often similar in family members, and also in successive generations within a family. There are, however, some important clues which suggest that an individual may be susceptible to cancer because of an inherited tendency. These clues will now be described.

Cancer in a near family member

Cancer diagnosed in a near relative is the most important first clue that a person may be prone to inherited cancer.

The parts of the body in which an inherited tendency appears to be important are the colon, rectum, breast and skin. It is also possible but less common to inherit a tendency for cancers in other parts of the body, particularly the uterus, ovary, lung, prostate, stomach and pancreas. Thus, if a close family member develops cancer in one of these parts of the body, this may be the first clue that others in the close family are also prone to cancer at that site due to an inherited tendency.

Other clues from the family history

Apart from a close family member developing a cancer, there are some other clues in the family history which would raise suspicion that there may be an inherited tendency for cancer.

- *Total number in the family with cancer.* If two or more members of the family develop cancer, and particularly if the cancer is in the same part of the body, such as the colon, rectum or breast.

- *Age at which cancer has developed.* If the cancer has developed at an earlier age than is usual for that cancer in the rest of the community.
- *Cancer in several generations.* If the cancer was present in a particular part of the body, such as the breast or the colon in successive generations.

ACTION TO TAKE IF INHERITED CANCER IS SUSPECTED

If inherited cancer is suspected, the first step is to get detailed information on the family history of cancer. To do this, Table 4.2, which appears at the end of this chapter, may be useful.

Importantly, it is necessary to find out if the members of the family did in fact develop cancer. If so, at what age, and whether they died from this condition. If they are alive then it is possible to find out from the family member exactly what type of cancer it is, and at what age it was identified. If they have died, it is often a good idea to obtain either a copy of the death certificate or talk to the treating doctor, as frequently the recollection of other family members may be hazy or inaccurate.

If there are characteristics in the family such as one or more cancers in near relatives, cancers in similar sites and over more than one generation, and cancers appearing at a relatively young age, then it is a good plan to draw a *family tree* identifying those who have had cancer, and whether they are alive or dead. A hypothetical family tree is shown in Figure 3. Based on this hypothetical situation, it can be seen that in this family there appears to be an inherited tendency for colorectal cancer on one side of the family, and of breast cancer on the other side of the family.

Figure 3: A 'family tree' of cancer in a hypothetical family

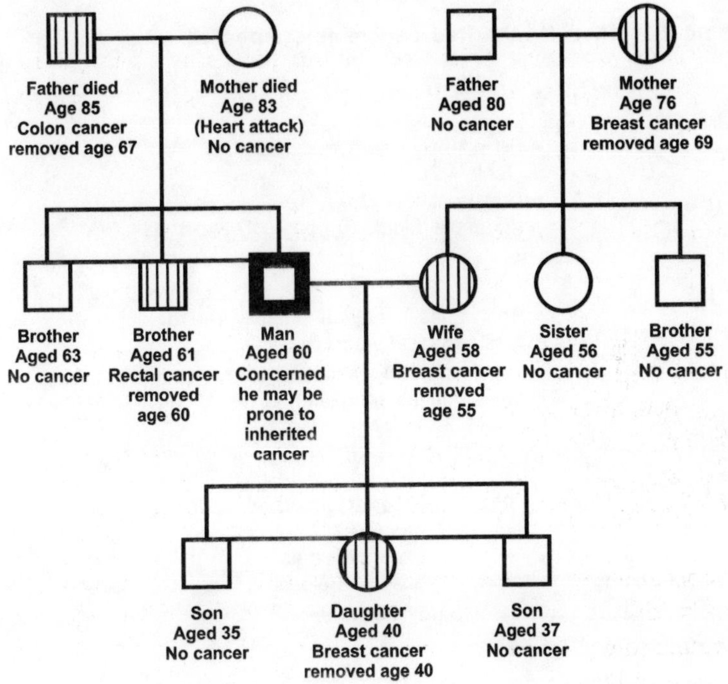

Father died
Age 85
Colon cancer
removed age 67

Mother died
Age 83
(Heart attack)
No cancer

Father
Aged 80
No cancer

Mother
Age 76
Breast cancer
removed age 69

Brother
Aged 63
No cancer

Brother
Aged 61
Rectal cancer
removed
age 60

Man
Aged 60
Concerned
he may be
prone to
inherited
cancer

Wife
Aged 58
Breast cancer
removed
age 55

Sister
Aged 56
No cancer

Brother
Aged 55
No cancer

Son
Aged 35
No cancer

Daughter
Aged 40
Breast cancer
removed age 40

Son
Aged 37
No cancer

The next step would be to present this information to one's medical practitioner who could then advise whether it is necessary to go to a centre for specialised genetic counselling, or whether it is more appropriate to be seen by particular experts regarding the need to be screened for an early cancer or a precancerous condition, or whether the medical practitioner is happy to pursue total care. Whatever option is chosen—to go to a centre for genetic counselling, or to attend a particular medical or surgical specialist, or for the general practitioner to handle the situation totally—it will be necessary to have a medical examination and possibly also to have certain screening tests performed. Based on the results of these tests, further treatment may or may not be necessary. After screening tests

Table 4.1: Plan if inherited cancer is suspected

1. • Fill in family history questionnaire
   (Table 4.2)
   • Construct family tree
   (Example, Figure 3)

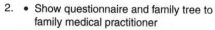

2. • Show questionnaire and family tree to
   family medical practitioner
   • Family medical practitioner will suggest
   one of the following alternatives:

3A. Family medical   **or**   3B. Referral to medical   **or**   3C. Referral to
    practitioner   or surgical   genetic
    continues with   expert, such as   counselling
    total care   gastroentrologist   centre
                                        or gynaecologist

4. Medical examination and screening tests,
   such as mammography, occult blood in
   the stool etc may be required

5. If screening and other tests are positive for
   cancer or precancerous conditions, appropriate
   treatment, such as removal of an early cancer or
   breast lump, skin mole etc may be needed

6. Subsequently the person may be advised to undergo
   further regular follow-up examinations or tests

have been performed and appropriate advice or treatment given, it may be necessary to return at regular intervals for further consultation and possibly for further tests. If inherited cancer is suspected, the wisest policy is to pursue the above plan of action, which is summarised in Table 4.1.

If a known inherited family cancer syndrome is present or strongly suspected, or if an inherited tendency for cancer which does not belong to a family cancer syndrome is suspected, then positive steps can be taken to confirm or refute this possibility. If inherited cancer is known to be present or if it is a possibility, then there are excellent means of identifying such cancers or precancerous conditions early, and removing them at a curable stage. The plan for identifying inherited cancer has been described in this chapter. It will also be emphasised in subsequent chapters when considering individual malignant tumours in those parts of the body in which an inherited tendency is a possibility.

Table 4.2: Family history of cancer

Relative concerned	Name	Year of birth	Is there a history of cancer? Write 'yes' or 'no' or 'don't know'	If yes, where is the cancer (such as breast, colon, rectum etc)?	Age cancer was found	Relative alive or dead	If dead, cause of death	If dead, was cause of death verified? Write Yes—doctor or Yes—death certificate, or No
Mother								
Father								
Sister								
Sister								
Sister								
Brother								
Brother								
Brother								
Child								
Child								
Child								
M/mother								
M/father								
F/mother								

Table 4.2 Family history of cancer (cont.)

Relative concerned	Name	Year of birth	Is there a history of cancer? Write 'yes' or 'no' or 'don't know'	If yes, where is the cancer (such as breast, colon, rectum etc)?	Age cancer was found	Relative alive or dead	If dead, cause of death	If dead, was cause of death verified? Write Yes—doctor or Yes—death certificate, or No
F/father								
M/sister								
M/sister								
M/sister								
M/brother								
M/brother								
M/brother								
F/sister								
F/sister								
F/sister								
F/brother								
F/brother								
F/brother								

5

Diet

An essential part of our human heritage is that we have a stomach and an appetite, and that we cannot forget about food for more than a few hours. The folklore and myth which surrounds food is almost endless, so we must be both careful and wise when advising entire populations regarding their dietary habits.

In developed Western countries, such as the USA, United Kingdom or Australia, one cancer in three is probably preventable by dietary change.

44

Cancer of the large bowel, that is colon or rectal cancer, as well as their precancerous conditions, colorectal adenomas, have an important dietary cause (Chapter 14). Diet is also likely to be a contributory cause of breast, prostate, stomach (gastric), gullet (oesophagus), uterine, ovarian, lung and cervix cancer (Table 5.1).

Table 5.1: Diet-related cancers

Diet a proven cause	Diet a likely contributory cause
Colon cancer	Breast cancer
Rectal cancer	Prostate cancer
Adenomatous polyps of colon and	Stomach (gastric) cancer
rectum (precancerous tumours)	Gullet (oesophagus) cancer
	Pancreas cancer
	Uterine cancer
	Ovarian cancer
	Lung cancer
	Cervix cancer

This chapter relates entirely to dietary recommendations which are appropriate for the prevention of a malignant tumour, and not for its treatment. There is an important difference between a diet recommended for the prevention of cancer and diets which have been recommended for the treatment of a cancer. The risk of developing diet-related cancers can be lowered by a certain type of diet, but so far there is little evidence that this same diet is useful in the treatment of a cancer once it has become established.

Almost nothing was known about the dietary prevention of cancer 30 years ago, but since that time enormous progress has been made in understanding the dietary causes of several cancers. The basic building blocks of a cancer prevention diet are now known. There is also new information constantly becoming available through research, which will continue to fine-tune the details of what is an appropriate diet.

> *The diet recommended for preventing cancer is similar for all the diet-related cancers, and it also happens to be similar to that recommended for the prevention of other common illnesses, in particular heart disease, narrowing of the arteries, and the type of diabetes which first appears in adult life. It is also the diet advocated for the maintenance of good health and vitality. This diet is nutritious, it can be made delicious and tasty, and it certainly need not be dull, tasteless or monotonous.*

Those aspects of diet which increase a person's risk of developing a cancer are first described, and then this is contrasted with the recommended cancer prevention diet. When describing the cancer prevention diet, a broad plan is first presented, then a practical menu with several substitutions is shown, followed by some suggestions for dietary change, practical tips for changing diet habit, as well as suggestions which may help in certain special situations away from home, such as while on holidays or when eating in restaurants. The role of nutritional supplements in a cancer prevention diet, such as vitamins and minerals, will also be described.

WHAT A CANCER-PRODUCING DIET IS

The main elements of an *undesirable* diet are summarised in Table 5.2.

Table 5.2: Elements of an undesirable diet

Calories: energy-rich foods, especially fats and sugars.
Fat: especially fats of animal origin, such as butter and lard.
Meat: especially beef, veal, lamb, and pork with fat on it. Smoked and cured meat such as bacon, and processed meat such as salami. Heavily fried and heavily grilled meat.
Salt: excessive added salt may contribute to some cancers.

Too many calories

*The lunches of fifty-seven years
had caused his chest to slip down
into the mezzanine floor.*

P.G. *Wodehouse (1881–1975)*

Eating a lot of energy-rich foods, being overweight, or both, raises the chances of developing many cancers, including cancers of the colon, rectum, breast, prostate, kidney, uterus, ovary and gallbladder. Energy-rich foods appear to be cancer-promoting because they may increase the rate at which cells in the body multiply, and perhaps also because cancer-producing agents are stored in the excess fat rather than eliminated in the urine or bowel motions; there are probably also other reasons which at present are unclear. Desirable weight for height can be checked from Table 5.3. Note that to a small extent weight depends on whether the body frame is small, average or large, and also that a person is still considered to be healthy if their actual weight is 10% more or 10% less than the figures shown in the table.

Table 5.3: Table of desirable weight for height

Women				Men			
cm	kg	ft in	lbs	cm	kg	ft in	lbs
148	49	4 10	108	155	56	5 1	124
150	50	4 11	111	158	58	5 2	128
153	52	5 0	114	160	59	5 3	130
155	53	5 1	117	163	60	5 4	133
158	54	5 2	120	165	62	5 5	137
160	56	5 3	124	168	64	5 6	141
163	58	5 4	128	170	66	5 7	146
165	60	5 5	133	173	68	5 8	150
168	62	5 6	137	175	69	5 9	153
170	63	5 7	139	178	72	5 10	158
173	65	5 8	143	180	74	5 11	163
175	67	5 9	148	183	76	6 0	167
178	69	5 10	153	185	78	6 1	172
180	70	5 11	155	188	80	6 2	176
183	72	6 0	158	190	82	6 3	180

Commonly eaten energy-rich foods are those containing simple sugars, such as sugar, ice-cream, some highly sugared cereals, lollies, many soft drinks, jam, marmalade and cakes. Fats, as present in butter, margarine, lard and various oils are even more energy-rich than are sugars. Some oils, such as olive oil, may protect against cancers. However, if a large quantity of oil is consumed, then the calories in the oil could do harm, cancelling out its beneficial effects. Remember that each gram of sugar produces 4 calories when used by the body, and each gram of fat produces 9 calories.

Too much fat

Fats are energy-rich. They contribute to heart disease, raise cholesterol levels, increase weight, and some fats also increase the risk of cancers of the colon, rectum, breast, ovary, uterus and prostate. This is particularly so for *saturated fats* which are found mainly in foods of animal origin (particularly in foods like butter, whole fat dairy products, such as milk, cream and cheese, in meat, chicken and eggs), and are also found in nuts and some oils, especially coconut oil. *Polyunsaturated fats* are found in some vegetable oils such as corn, sesame, sunflower, maize, soy bean and safflower oil, and they may not be as great a risk as saturated fats. However, polyunsaturated fats are also full of energy and their consumption is best kept to a minimum. *Mono-unsaturated fats* are found in olive oil, peanut oil and canola oil, and in general are regarded as a good choice of fat, and may even be useful in the prevention of some cancers. However, it should be remembered that in common with other types of fats, eating large amounts of mono-unsaturated fats has the disadvantage of consuming too many calories.

The high fat content of some foods is often not appreciated, and we call this *hidden fat*. To be remembered in this category are salad dressings, nuts and seeds, biscuits, chips and crackers, peanut butter, creamy soups, preserved meats and processed meats such as sausages, hamburgers and salami.

Although it is not precisely known how fats promote the growth of some cancers, they do appear to produce free radicals in the body which can damage DNA, leading to mutations in the dividing cells. Fats can increase the rate of cell division in the body, putting it into 'metabolic overdrive', thereby increasing the chances of mutations. Fats can also interfere with the part of the immune system that normally destroys cancer cells. Finally, fat cells can concentrate and store certain carcinogens, such as pesticides, and also some hormones, such as oestrogens.

Too much meat

> When mighty roast beef
> was the Englishman's food,
> It ennobled our hearts and enriched our blood.
> [with fat and heterocyclic amines—author]

> The Roast Beef of England
> Richard Leveridge (1670–1758)

Too much meat is harmful, partly because it often contains too much fat, partly because it contains some cancer-producing substances, and partly because frying and grilling can produce substances which damage the DNA in dividing human cells, giving rise to abnormal or 'dysplastic' cells, and partly because cancer-producing *nitrosamines* and other carcinogenic substances, such as dioxin, may be present in meat. Heavily fried and grilled meat, as well as fried and grilled chicken also contains several chemicals, including compounds called *heterocyclic amines*, which can damage the DNA in cells. Consumption of preserved, smoked or cured meat, and probably also smoked or cured fish or chicken and pickled foods of all types, produces carcinogenic substances, such as nitrosamines and sulphides. These foods should be eaten in small quantities or not at all.

Excessive added salt

Excessive added salt may contribute to stomach, colon and rectal cancers, for reasons that at present are not clear. The high salt content of some foods is often forgotten. There is 'hidden salt' in soya and other sauces, potato chips, hamburgers, other take-away foods, processed foods, salted nuts, pickled food and even in beer. It has been estimated that only about one-quarter of the salt content in an average Western diet is added by the consumer and three-quarters is hidden salt contained in processed foods.

WHAT A CANCER PREVENTION DIET IS

> *Fight Cancer with the Help*
> *of your Greengrocer.*
>
> *Headline in* The Age, *1994*

The foods which form a cancer prevention diet are shown in Table 5.4. In the main these are foods of plant origin, particularly vegetables, fruit and cereals, all of which contain dietary fibre, and also contain many other beneficial substances. Also important in this cancer prevention diet are starch-rich foods, such as bread, pasta and rice, as well as fish. Lean meat, skinless poultry and fat-reduced or fat-free dairy foods can also be eaten.

- *Vegetables.* All types of vegetables are by far the most important foods in a cancer prevention diet. Many vegetables have strong anticancer properties, especially cruciferous vegetables (cabbage, cauliflower, broccoli, brussel sprouts, kohlrabi, swede, turnip, kale), garlic, onions and chives, leafy green vegetables, carrots, pumpkin and tomatoes. These vegetables contain compounds which have anticancer properties and have been collectively called *phytochemicals*. These phytochemicals include beta-carotene, vitamins C and E, which are antioxidants, lycopene—a strong antioxidant and a strong inhibitor of cell multiplication found in tomatoes—as well as several other compounds, including

Table 5.4: Elements of an anticancer diet

1. Vegetables, vegetables, vegetables
2. Fruits
3. Cereals
4. Starchy foods, such as bread, pasta and rice
5. Fish of all types
6. Low-fat or non-fat dairy foods, such as low-fat milk, skim milk, low-fat yoghurt, low-fat cottage cheese
7. Skinless poultry and lean meat occasionally

folic acid, indoles, linolenic acid, dithiolthiones, genistein, tannins and isothiocyanates. There are probably numerous other protective compounds present in vegetables which have not even been identified so far. These compounds act in many ways because of their several anticancer properties, which include action as antioxidants, inhibitors of cancer-producing nitrosamines, and regulators of normal cell division, cell maturation and cell death.

- *Fruits*. These contain vitamin C, beta-carotene and other compounds with anticancer properties, such as flavonoids, limonoids and others. Raspberries and strawberries contain tannins and recent research suggests that these compounds may be protective against cancer of the cervix, and possibly other cancers also.

- *Cereals*. Grains and cereals contain complex sugars and starches, vitamin E, folic acid, minerals like selenium and magnesium, linolenic acid, phenolic acids and precursors of vitamin D, compounds which have all been shown to have anticancer properties.

- *Dietary fibre*. The undigestible part of vegetables, fruits and cereals contains numerous substances which are collectively called *dietary fibre*. Dietary fibre confers protection against certain cancers, particularly cancers of the colon and rectum, and possibly also against other cancers, such as breast and prostate cancer. It does this in several ways, which includes diluting carcinogens in food, and by producing short chain fatty acids in the bowel, especially *butyrate*, which has anticancer properties.

- *Starch-rich foods*. These include bread, pasta and rice. Brown (wholegrain) rice is preferable to white rice. Starches have anticancer properties for reasons similar to dietary fibre. They also produce short chain fatty acids in the bowel which may help in the prevention of bowel cancer and probably of other cancers also.

- *Fish.* All fish is low in saturated fat, and contains special fats called omega–3 fatty acids (fish oil), which has been shown to have anticancer properties, particularly for cancers of the colon, rectum, breast, prostate, ovary and uterus. Fish also contains selenium and other compounds which may have anticancer effects.

Anticancer vitamins and minerals in food

Throughout this book reference will be made to vitamin-containing foods, and to minerals such as selenium, in the dietary prevention of various cancers. The following is a *selection* of foods (not a complete list) which contain an abundant supply of the vitamins and minerals which appear to be relevant in cancer prevention.

- *Beta-carotene (provitamin A).* Carrots, spinach, broccoli, pumpkin, apricots, peaches, cantaloup, mango.
- *Vitamin C.* Oranges, lemons, currents, most other fruits, peppers, parsley, cabbage, cauliflower, broccoli, spinach.
- *Vitamin E.* Peanuts, almonds, peanut butter, wheat bran, wheat-germ, sweet potato, spinach, vegetable oils.
- *Folic acid (folate, folacin).* Liver, especially chicken liver, wheat bran, baker's yeast (bread), spinach, cabbage, cauliflower, broccoli, endive, peanuts, peanut butter.
- *Selenium.* Fish, cereals, garlic.
- *Calcium.* Milk, skim milk, cheese, cottage cheese, yoghurt (use low-fat or no-fat varieties in a cancer prevention diet).

RECOMMENDED DIET

For many, changing eating habits will be one of the most difficult things to achieve in a cancer prevention programme. At the same time, dietary change is likely to be the most rewarding. Research suggests that a person is never too old to change dietary habits and still receive protection in relation to diet-related illnesses. A personal interest in cooking and in the taste of food, as well as an understanding of what nutrients different foods contain, are likely to be positive factors for dietary change. The diet recommended below will not only lower cancer risk, but will also decrease weight in those who are overweight, and help in the prevention of heart disease, as well as help to maintain sound health and a vigorous lifestyle. The general principles of a cancer prevention diet are indicated in Table 5.5.

Table 5.5: Cancer prevention diet—general principles

The main constituents of the cancer prevention diet.
(This diet is also useful for preventing heart and blood vessel disease, adult-onset diabetes and for the maintenance of good health.)

1. Total calories not to exceed 2500 calories per day for most men and 2000 calories for most women. More calories are allowable for those doing strenuous physical work or strenuous physical activity each day, and less for older adults who are not particularly active.
2. Eat plenty of vegetables, bread, pasta, rice, cereals and fruit.
3. Reduce the fat in your diet to 20% of total daily calories. How this important part of your diet can be achieved will be illustrated by example shortly in the food pyramid and in the cancer prevention menu.
4. Eat fish regularly.
5. Eat small amounts of lean meat from which all visible fat has been removed.
6. Eat small amounts of skinless chicken.
7. Avoid heavily fried and heavily grilled meat, chicken or fish.
8. Eat low-fat or non-fat dairy products, such as low-fat or non-fat milk, skim milk, yoghurt, cottage cheese.
9. Eat little or no smoked, cured or preserved foods.
10. Avoid excessive added salt in cooking and in all processed foods, and eat little or no salted or pickled foods.

THE FOOD PYRAMID CHART

A food pyramid chart has been produced by the US Department of Agriculture and Department of Health and Human Services.

It is often used in a modified form by many similar agencies in numerous countries. This chart, reproduced in a modified form in Figure 4, provides a simple guide to how much of each main food group one should eat in a healthy diet, including the daily number of servings of each. The size of the servings in the food pyramid is indicated in Table 5.6.

Figure 4: The food pyramid

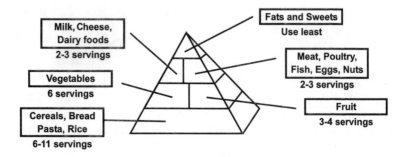

Table 5.6: Size of servings in food pyramid

Food	Size of one serving
Bread	1 slice
Pasta	½ cup of cooked pasta
Rice	½ cup of cooked rice
Cereal	1 cup of cold ready-to-eat cereal *or* ½ cup of cooked cereal
Vegetable	½ cup of cooked or raw vegetables *or* 1 cup of leafy vegetables
Fruit	1 piece of fruit or equivalent wedge of melon etc ½ cup canned/stewed fruit ¼ cup dried fruit
Low-fat milk	1 cup
Low-fat yoghurt	1 cup
Low-fat cottage cheese	¼ cup
Low-fat cheese	1 slice (50 g or 1½ ounces natural, 65 g or 2 ounces processed cheese)
Fish	100 g (3 ounces)
Lean meat or skinless chicken	100 g (3 ounces)
Egg	1 egg

The food pyramid chart is a good food guide, and we can now fine-tune this even more because of recent information. Recent studies suggest that we emphasise vegetables as the most important protective agent against cancers, followed by fruits, then cereals, pasta, rice and bread. Fish is increasingly being emphasised as protective against several cancers. It is best to consume low-fat or non-fat milk products. Lean meat and skinless poultry can be eaten in small quantities, whilst fats and sweets should be eaten least of all.

A CANCER PREVENTION MENU

Table 5.7 provides a more accurate idea of the type of menu which is useful in a cancer prevention diet. This menu would be almost identical to a diet which is recommended for the prevention of heart disease, adult-onset diabetes and for the maintenance of vigorous good health.

The menu in Table 5.7 should be regarded as a flexible guide, so that foods can be substituted, provided they are from the same food grouping, and the size of the serve is similar to that suggested. Also, any spices can be added to taste (with the exception of salt, which is best used sparingly). It is important to eat three meals every day. Never skip breakfast, usually an all plant food meal. Most of all, enjoy every meal.

Table 5.7: A cancer prevention menu

Meal	Typical food	Serve size	Typical alternatives, choose one item	Serve size
Breakfast	Fresh fruit	1 pce	• Canned fruit • Stewed fruit • Dried fruit • Orange juice • Vegetable juice (no added sugar in juices)	½ cup ½ cup ¼ cup ½ cup ½ cup
	Cold wheat/bran cereal Low-fat milk or low-fat yoghurt	1 cup 1 cup	• Porridge/oatmeal • Wholemeal toast • Wholemeal/bran bun or roll • Wholemeal/bran crumpet/waffle • Once per week—eggs poached or scrambled	1 cup 2 sls 1 pce 2 pcs 2 eggs
	Tea, coffee	1 cup	• Cocoa, carob • Water	1 cup 1 cup
Lunch	Tomato juice	1 cup	• Grapefruit or other fruit juice • Vegetable juice • Mineral water • Water (no added sugar in juices)	1 cup 1 cup 1 cup 1 cup
	Tuna or other canned fish and salad sandwich, wholemeal bread (or similar) + raw vegetables (carrot, tomato, capsicum, celery etc)	2 sls 1–3	• Chicken, lean beef or turkey instead of tuna or canned fish • Low-fat cottage cheese + fruit (cut up fresh) + low-fat crackers/biscuits • Low-fat soup, no meat + wholemeal, rye or similar bread • Pizza, low-fat cheese, tomato, anchovies, olives (or similar)	1 sl ½ cup ½ cup 2 pcs 1 cup 2 sls 2 sls

Meal	Typical food	Serve size	Typical alternatives, choose one item	Serve size
	Fruit	1 pce or equiv	• Canned fruit (no added sugar)	½ cup
	Herbal tea/black/green tea	1 cup	• Iced tea • Mineral water • Ginger ale • Low calorie tonic water • Water	1 cup 1 cup 1 cup 1 cup 1 cup
Dinner	Baked, poached or lightly grilled fish (2–3 times per week)	100 g (3 oz) or one fillet	• Lean meat (1–2 per week) • Skinless chicken (1–2 per week) • Pasta and sauce • Pizza, low-fat cheese	100 g 100 g 1 cup 2 sls

(If having fish, about ½ your plate should be the fish and ½ vegetables and/or salad or grains. If having meat or chicken, 1/3 of plate should be lean meat/skinless chicken and 2/3 vegetables and/or salad or grains.)

Meal	Typical food	Serve size	Typical alternatives, choose one item	Serve size
	Steamed vegetables	1 cup	• Salad with low-fat dressing • Baked vegetables • Wholegrain rice, cous cous, polenta, or similar grains	2 cups 1 cup 1 cup
	Frozen low-fat yoghurt + fruit (no added sugar)	1 cup	• Fruit salad • Low-fat yoghurt • Stewed fruit • Jelly & fresh fruit	1 cup ½ cup 1 cup 1 cup
	Herbal tea/black/green tea	1 cup	• Mineral water • Wine	1 glass 1 glass
Snack	Fruit, fruit pieces, fruit salad	1 pce or 1 cup	• Low-fat or skim milk • Low-fat frozen yoghurt • Raw celery, capsicum, carrot, or other vegetables • Raisins, currants or dried fruit • Low-fat crackers • Low-fat biscuits	1 cup 1 cup 2 or more pcs ½ cup 2 pcs 2 pcs

A DOZEN SUGGESTIONS TO HELP CHANGE DIETARY HABITS

- *Take time over the change,* do it over a 2–3 month period. For the first 3–4 weeks write down what you eat and compare it to the food pyramid chart and to the cancer prevention menu described above.
- *Whenever possible, choose healthier alternatives,* such as steamed vegetables instead of fried vegetables, baked fish instead of fried fish, low-fat milk instead of full-cream milk.
- *Eat smaller portions* of meat and fatty foods, and eat little or no smoked, preserved, cured or pickled foods. Eat sausages and hamburgers infrequently.
- *Eat low-fat or non-fat dairy foods,* such as low-fat milk, cottage cheese, yoghurt, ice-cream or cheese.
- *Avoid deep frying or extensive frying.* Cooking methods which use little or no fat, such as steaming, poaching, baking and microwaving are preferable. Stir fry instead of frying in a lot of fat. Olive oil is generally more stable than other oils when heated. Use non-stick sprays in cooking utensils rather than fat. When grilling use a grid, avoid hot plates, and avoid charring the food.
- *Use suitable herbs, spices and seasoning* as their liberal and varied use gives food a variety of interesting tastes.
- *Use low-fat or non-fat dressings and sauces.* These taste just like their oily and fatty equivalents. Use salsa and other similar vegetable sauces for stews, as they usually contain no fat.
- *Eat a meatless main meal most days of the week.* Fish is not counted as meat.
- *Remove all visible fat from meat and all skin from poultry.* The meat and poultry taste will remain unchanged when the fat is removed.
- *Always look for foods low in fat or containing no fat,* such as vegetables, fruit, cereals, rice and pasta. Read food labels in shops and supermarkets and choose low-fat, low-energy alternatives. Plan your meals up to a week ahead, and

use *shopping lists* to avoid impulse buying of unhealthy alternatives.

- *Use health-oriented cookbooks.* Choose those cookbooks which emphasise low-fat, low meat, high vegetable, high fruit and high cereal and starch-containing dishes which are tasty and varied. There are now good cookbooks of this type available, such as *Julie Stafford's Taste of Life* (Penguin), *Rosemary Stanton's Gut Buster Recipes* (Allen & Unwin), and others. It should be possible to write your own cookbook within a short time of starting this menu! Also, developing an interest in the taste of food and in cooking adds to the motivation to eat tasty, healthy food.

- *If you have a medical problem, seek professional help.* For those who have a weight problem, or have a condition already requiring dietary treatment, such as diabetes, first discuss the cancer prevention diet with a dietitian or a medical practitioner.

CANCER PREVENTION DIET UNDER SPECIAL CIRCUMSTANCES

If you visit a restaurant, go to a take-away food outlet, eat at a friend's home, or travel on business or holiday, some difficulties may be encountered in sticking to the cancer prevention diet. If this occurs uncommonly, say one meal per week, then it should not pose a problem and the other two meals for that day can simply be readjusted to equalise. These are a few suggestions of how one might cope with these situations.

Restaurants

There are a number of ways of enjoying restaurant food and yet still keep close to a healthy diet. Make a habit of choosing food which is low in fat and calorie content and cooked with little or no fat, such as poached, steamed or baked food. Eat smaller portions, particularly of fatty or fried foods. Restaurants also provide a great opportunity to eat healthy foods which are more difficult to prepare at home, such as fish. Restaurants emphasising ethnic food, such as Greek, Italian, Chinese, Mexican, Middle Eastern, Japanese, Vietnamese and Indian, almost always have low-fat foods on their menus, with plenty of vegetables and many starch-rich foods. An occasional vegetarian meal for the non-vegetarian can be a novel and exciting experience, as can visits to these interesting ethnic restaurants. Sometimes the chef will prepare a healthy low-fat, low-energy alternative, or modify the main course on request. Eat salads, and ask for a dressing on the side so that the amount of dressing used can be controlled. Beware of dishes prepared with butter, margarine or cheese.

Take-away food

This can be difficult as the energy derived from the fat content of food in the usual hamburger and fried chicken chains is often about 50%. It's best to avoid these places, but if there is nowhere else, choose healthier alternatives such as salad, plain hamburgers, grilled or baked chicken rather than fried food. There are now also many take-away outlets with low-fat food, rice and vegetables, such as those which emphasise Asian, Japanese, Mexican, Middle Eastern or Indian foods. Small delicatessens serving fresh and healthy food containing a lot of vegetables and salads are becoming increasingly popular for lunches.

Eating at friends

This can be difficult because of the sensibilities of the cook and the pride with which food is prepared in many homes. It is often best to be frank and explain that you are trying to change your dietary habits and eat foods which contain less fat and fewer calories, to eat more vegetables, salads, fruit and fish, and eat less fat and meat. If this is difficult, it is always possible to eat a smaller portion. Remember that it is also possible to cut back on other food eaten on the day of the dinner, or make up for it later by cutting back over the next few days. It is interesting that most of my friends now know my changed dietary habits, and in fact some of them have also changed their eating habits as a result.

Travelling by plane

This is now quite simple, and even for short trips which involve a meal, it is possible to ask for a low-fat or vegetarian type of meal. However, remember that it is necessary to request this well before travelling. Interestingly, these special meals are often not only healthier, but are fresher and taste better than the standard airline meal.

Holidays

If it is a holiday in which most of the food is taken from home, then always choose the healthier low-calorie, low-fat alternatives which include lots of vegetables, fruit, cereals, bread, pasta and rice. If buying food to cook on holidays, always choose low-fat and low-energy foods such as fish, skinless chicken and lean meat. Use low-fat or non-fat dairy products and low-fat salad dressings. If staying in a guest house or hotel, use similar ploys to those used in a restaurant, by eating smaller portions, choosing healthier alternatives that are low in calories, low in fat and cooked with little or no fat.

Needing a 'binge'

'Everything in moderation, including moderation', is something I said irreverently at an international nutrition and cancer conference in 1975, and for me it still holds today. *Remember, it is what one usually eats, and not what one eats occasionally that matters most.* If circumstances are such that it is difficult to resist, or for some special reason a 'diet binge' is required, have it once in a while, enjoy it to the full, and cut back later!

VITAMINS, MINERALS AND OTHER NUTRITIONAL SUPPLEMENTS

Although vitamins, minerals and other nutritional supplements have long been advocated by enthusiasts for the prevention of many illnesses, including various cancers, the scientific evidence that they have a role in cancer prevention is quite limited. At present there is reasonable evidence that there *may* be a preventive role for multivitamin and mineral preparations (colon and rectal cancer), vitamin C supplements (colon and rectal cancer), vitamin E supplements (prostate cancer), garlic extract (colon and rectal cancer), fish oil supplements (colon and rectal cancer and adenoma, possibly breast cancer, prostate cancer and cancer of the uterus), and selenium (prostate cancer, colon and rectal cancer and adenoma). The term *chemoprevention* was coined in the 1970s by Dr Michael Sporn in the USA, for compounds used in the primary prevention of various cancers, often but not always as nutritional supplements. In several parts of this book you will read about this relatively new and potentially useful approach to the primary prevention of cancer.

- *I emphasise that it is the nutrients in the anticancer diet which are the most important part of any nutritional advice on cancer prevention.* It is greatly preferable to eat vitamins and minerals as whole foods, rather than taking them as nutritional supplements. Nutritional supplements such as vitamins or minerals are probably only useful in certain situations. Extra vitamins and minerals over and above those supplied in a healthy diet may be necessary during pregnancy, after an illness, or with excessive life stresses. However, it is important to understand that nutritional supplements are not the 'quick fix' for those who eat an unhealthy diet, smoke, do no exercise and drink excessive amounts of alcohol.

- *Supplemental vitamins and minerals in recommended small doses can probably do no harm, and there is some limited evidence that in certain individuals at higher than average risk of developing certain cancers, their risk may be lowered.* Individuals may be at high risk for certain cancers because of poor dietary habit, smoking or excessive alcohol consumption, and supplemental vitamin and mineral use in small doses *may* decrease their chances of developing cancers of the colon, rectum, breast, prostate and possibly uterus and ovary, although this has not been proven. The regular use of a moderate dose multivitamin and mineral preparation, which includes vitamin C, vitamin E and folic acid, freely available over the counter, seems a reasonable though so far unproven tactic. Additionally, the daily use of relatively small doses of *vitamin C* (about 500–1000 mg per day), *vitamin E* (about 500 units per day), *fish oil containing omega–3 fatty acids* (about 400 mg of fatty acids), *odourless garlic extract* (about 500 mg of fresh bulb equivalent), and *selenium* (50–200 micrograms), is unlikely to do harm and may be of some protective value, especially among those at higher than average risk of developing cancers of the colon, rectum, breast, prostate, and possibly uterus and ovary. If you are in any doubt about the use of supplements, discuss it with your doctor first.

- *Recent reports are confusing regarding the role of beta-carotene supplements.* Until there is further scientific evidence, it would be best not to use beta-carotene supplements, and concentrate more on foods in your diet that contain beta-carotene, such as carrots, pumpkin, parsley, spinach, broccoli, endive and sweet potato, and fruits such as apricots, cantaloup, peach and mango.

- *Several other nutritional supplements have been described as possibly useful in cancer prevention.* These include soy bean extracts, soya products such as *bean curd (tofu)*, *ellagic acid* extracted from raspberries or strawberries, *indoles* from cruciferous vegetables, and others such as *brewed green tea*, and we eagerly await the results of scientific studies of their effectiveness in preventing cancers. The cancers targeted for prevention with the use of these compounds include cancers of the breast, colon, rectum, prostate, cervix and skin.

- *Pharmaceutical products* such as *tamoxifen* to prevent breast cancer and *finasteride* to prevent prostate cancer, and several others, are also being tested at present in scientific trials.

SPECIAL ANTICANCER DIETS

There are many so-called 'special anticancer diets' advocated by enthusiasts. It is most important to understand that most of these are advised as part of the treatment of an established cancer, and not for its prevention. This book deals entirely with the prevention and early detection of cancers. The treatment of an established cancer is outside the scope of this book.

Vegetarian diet

There is a spectrum of vegetarian diets of various grades and severity, and a full discussion of these diets will not be presented here. As a general principle, vegetarian diets are known to lower the risk of cancer in general, and of diet-related cancers in particular, such as cancers of the colon and rectum and some others. It has also been found that vegetarians are about 40% less likely to die of cancer than are non-vegetarians.

Vegetarians often lead a healthy lifestyle, in that many are non-smokers, avoid excessive alcohol, and keep fit with regular physical activity. They also often reduce their stress levels by meditation, relaxation and other similar techniques. Vegetarian diets are a reasonable alternative to the cancer prevention diet described above, and particularly so if the individual also avoids smoking and excessive alcohol consumption, performs physical activity regularly, and also uses methods of stress reduction such as meditation. *If you wish to start or pursue a vegetarian diet, discuss this with a medical practitioner first, to be certain that the proposed diet contains sufficient calories, protein, and essential fatty acids, as well as essential amino acids, vitamins and minerals.*

Macrobiotic diet

This has been used for the treatment of established cancers, and it has also been advocated as a type of diet suitable for the prevention of illness in general, including cancer. Although there are various grades of macrobiotic diet, the advocates of this diet believe that approximately half the diet should consist of whole grains, a further quarter of vegetables and the remainder of soups, beans, bean products and seaweeds. While meat, chicken, eggs and dairy products are not part of this diet, it can include the occasional use of white meat, fish, fruit and sweets. As with vegetarianism, in principle this is a low-fat, low calorie, high-fibre, high plant food diet, and would be reasonable for cancer prevention when practised in one of its moderate forms. However, extreme forms of macrobiotic diets can lead to calorie deficiency as well as to dangerously low intakes of protein, essential fatty acids, essential amino acids, and some vitamins and minerals. Some macrobiotic diets include water restriction, which is dangerous at all ages and especially so in the elderly. *If you wish to start or pursue a macrobiotic type of diet, discuss it first with a medical practitioner.*

'Alternative' diets

These have been mainly advocated as an additional form of treatment of an established cancer rather than for cancer prevention. These diets include dietary supplements, enzymes, liquid diets, huge doses of vitamins, or herbal treatments in which the composition of the nutritional supplement is often unclear. In others there is a diet as well as the use of special enemas. *I would like to discourage the use of these types of extreme diets, as well as the use of extreme forms of dietary* supplements, because they are totally inappropriate as part of a cancer prevention programme.

FINAL RECOMMENDATIONS

- *The essentials of a cancer prevention diet* are that it is very high in vegetables, high in fruit, cereals and starch-rich foods such as bread, pasta and rice, and is also high in fish. The diet should be low in fat, sugars and calories. Make sure that you eat lean meat and skinless poultry in small quantities and that you eat or drink low-fat or non-fat dairy foods, avoid excessive added salt, and eat little or no smoked, cured or pickled foods. Use healthy cooking methods whenever possible, such as steaming, boiling, poaching, microwaving or wok-frying. A high intake of calories, fat, sugar or meat should be avoided whenever possible.
- *The food pyramid chart is a good general guide.*
- *The cancer prevention menu* provides a basis for particular foods, and the information given in this book can be used to further develop and refine it to individual taste.
- *Useful suggestions about diet change* and how dietary habits can be altered to eat a healthy and enjoyable diet are also presented.
- *Suggestions for special situations,* such as eating in restaurants, with friends, or whilst on holidays are presented.
- *Nutritional supplements of vitamins, minerals and other supplements* can be a useful adjunct in cancer prevention under certain circumstances, and when used in small doses, but remember that it is the cancer prevention diet itself which is the most important.
- *Avoid so-called special 'alternative' diets* because of the risk of developing malnutrition and nutritional deficiencies. Moderate forms of vegetarian diets, or moderate forms of a so-called macrobiotic diet are reasonable, always provided they are nutritionally sound with regard to calories, protein, essential fatty acids, essential amino acids, vitamins and

minerals, including trace elements, and provided that it has been checked by a medical practitioner first to be sure that it is suitable for the individual in question.

- *Enjoy eating interesting, tasty and healthy food!*

6

Tobacco

It has been estimated that almost one cancer in three is smoking related.

It was a dramatic suggestion in 1950 by Dr Ernst Wynder and colleagues in New York, followed a few months later by Sir Richard Doll and Sir Austin Bradford Hill in London (then Drs Richard Doll and Austin Bradford Hill), that tobacco use is an important cause of lung cancer. The results of their scientific studies were ground-breaking in the history of cancer prevention. Very quickly, other researchers around the world confirmed that smoking is the most important single cause of lung cancer, and by the mid–1960s this was scientifically proven and almost universally accepted. Subsequently, researchers also found smoking to be an important cause in less commonly seen cancers, such as cancers of the mouth, throat and gullet (oesophagus), and it was suspected to be a cancer cause in other parts of the body also.

Why smoking is unhealthy

> *Tobacco drieth the brain, dimmeth the sight,*
> *hurteth the stomach, disturbeth the humors and spirits,*
> *corrupteth the breath, induceth a trembling of the limbs,*
> *exciteth the windpipe and lungs, scorcheth the heart and*
> *causes the blood to be thickened.*

> The Road to a Long Healthy Life
> *Tobias Venner (1577–1660)*

It has been shown beyond doubt that half of all regular smokers die prematurely from a smoking-related disease. Tobacco use causes lung cancer, which is the first or second cause of cancer death in most developed countries. It causes cancers in other parts of the body also, and if this isn't enough, it is also one of the important causes of heart attacks, emphysema, chronic bronchitis and other chronic lung conditions. Smoking also narrows blood vessels in the body and is responsible for major circulation problems in the legs, resulting in pain, gangrene and leg amputation. It promotes tooth and gum problems and peptic ulcers.

The illnesses and deaths caused by smoking are quite well known to the general public, so why is it that in many Western countries about one in four of the adult population over 18 still smoke? At least one important reason is that tobacco is a highly addictive habit.

Why smoking is bad for your family and the community

Smoking costs every community enormous sums of money in health bills, equally enormous sums of money in loss of productivity because of sick days, and therefore these aspects of smoking are harmful to the economy of the whole community and country.

Smokers are a danger to others around them who inhale their tobacco smoke. Mothers who smoke during pregnancy pass on to the child in their womb some harmful products of tobacco through the blood stream and placenta. Smoking can increase the chance of a miscarriage or stillbirth, and these mothers can produce unhealthy babies with a low birth weight. Moreover, the chances of children smoking when they grow up is increased if the parents smoke also. Childhood asthma is more common in families where the parents smoke. Smoking and tobacco use have devastating effects, not only on the individual, but also on the smoker's family, friends and on the whole community, and therefore smoking can no longer be regarded as a personal and private habit.

One of the problems about the ill-effects of smoking is that most individuals who become regular smokers commence smoking as teenagers and at a time when they are otherwise in excellent health, and when thoughts of dying are not on their minds. Moreover, the effects of tobacco use usually don't come to the forefront for 20 or 30 years after commencing smoking. There are a few who develop ill-health, such as severe bronchitis or asthma early in their smoking career, and some of these individuals are smart enough to recognise the warning signs and give up the habit before chronic smoking-related ill-health becomes apparent.

WHERE, WHY AND HOW SMOKING CAUSES CANCER

Lung cancer is the first or second most important cause of death from cancer in developed countries. Smoking is the important cause in five of six new lung cancers, in two of three mouth and throat cancers, in half of all gullet (oesophagus) cancers, and in one of three kidney, pancreas and urinary bladder cancers (Table 6.1).

Why does smoking produce cancers in the lung, mouth, throat,

Table 6.1: Smoking-related cancers

Smoking a proven cause	Smoking a likely contributory cause	Smoking a possible contributory cause
Lung cancer	Stomach (gastric) cancer	Colon cancer
Mouth cancer	Kidney cancer	Rectal cancer
Throat cancer	Cervix cancer	Primary liver cancer
Gullet (oesophagus) cancer	Colon adenomas (polyps)	Prostate cancer
Bladder cancer	Rectal adenomas (polyps)	Penis cancer
Pancreas cancer	Anal cancer	

gullet and elsewhere? The International Agency for Research on Cancer, a part of the World Health Organisation, has collected information which shows that there are over 4000 compounds in tobacco and tobacco smoke, and of these, at least 50 are carcinogenic and promote cancer. Cancer promotion in the lung, mouth, throat and gullet probably occurs to a large extent as a result of contact of the lining of the lung, mouth and throat with tobacco and tobacco smoke. It causes damage in various ways, including damage to the DNA of the dividing lining cells. Over the years, and occurring in several steps, the normal lining cell is changed to a cell which more and more resembles a cancer cell. Eventually the DNA is further damaged, so that it becomes an actual cancer cell which escapes the normal control of the body, and develops into a cancer which can grow and spread, and if unchecked, can kill the individual. Moreover, some cancer-producing chemicals in tobacco smoke enter the circulation in the lung, and are carried around the body by the blood stream, promoting cancer in parts of the body far removed from the mouth, throat and lungs, in organs such as the pancreas, kidneys and urinary bladder.

PREVENTING SMOKING-RELATED CANCERS

There is convincing scientific evidence that non-smokers are at a very low risk of developing cancers in which tobacco use is an important cause, such as cancers of the lung, mouth, throat and gullet. There is also excellent evidence that those who have been longstanding regular smokers can considerably decrease their chances of developing a smoking-related cancer if they quit and remain non-smokers thereafter. Obviously the best way of preventing smoking-related cancers, and other smoking-related illnesses is to not smoke at all. There is good evidence that a philosophy of non-smoking is best taught early in life, preferably in primary school, as well as by parental example. The next best is to quit smoking after this unhealthy habit has been started.

About one of every five smokers seems to be able to give up the smoking habit without any major difficulties. Those who can stop smoking easily are often not heavy smokers, and often an important health event had occurred in their lives or in the lives of their friends, such as when a member of the family who is a smoker develops lung cancer. For the other four of five smokers, or in 80% of all established smokers, it is difficult to give up smoking. We will now examine the reasons for this more closely, because they are important in determining the best ways to quit.

Why is quitting difficult?

Smoke, smoke, smoke that cigarette
Puff, puff, puff and if you puff yourself to death
Tell St Peter at the Golden Gate
That you just hate to make him wait
But you just gotta have another cigarette.

Merle Davis and Tex Williams

Addiction

For many years tobacco companies have denied that tobacco use is addictive, in spite of sound and convincing evidence to the contrary. It is probably the nicotine in the tobacco and tobacco smoke which is responsible for the person having a temporary feeling of elation and it is probably this feeling which results in an addiction. This feeling of elation is very temporary, and it can cause withdrawal symptoms when nicotine disappears from the blood stream. Withdrawal symptoms in heavy smokers include a feeling of tiredness and drowsiness, poor sleep, a dry mouth and a general lack of energy. Withdrawal of nicotine can also result in a person becoming irritable and anxious without an obvious reason for this behaviour.

Friends and circumstances

At least one of the disturbing trends among teenage men and women who smoke is that their friends are smoking also, and that it gives them a feeling of control over their lives in relation to the 'adult community'. Smoking thus becomes a social statement, albeit very misdirected, because eventually most of the harm is to the individual who smokes and not to the community.

Stress

Life stresses, such as the demands of work, the problems of family life, money problems, and even social encounters, can be extremely stressful to individuals. One of the ways of combating these stresses is to smoke and get a 'nicotine buzz' to help deal with these life stresses.

A QUIT SMOKING PROGRAMME

There is no foolproof or best way to quit smoking, although some methods suit a certain group of smokers better than others. It is not uncommon for an individual to try more than one method, since quitting smoking is often a 'trial and error' process.

Complete withdrawal

This method is sometimes referred to as *cold turkey*, and it is a sudden and complete cessation of smoking and tobacco use. This is often successful with those who have not been very heavy smokers, and not over a long period of time, such as someone smoking 10–15 cigarettes per day for about ten years.

When using this method, it is important to pay attention to withdrawal symptoms, and handle them as they arise. Irritability and a feeling of anxiety can often be combated by gentle physical activity such as walking, swimming or cycling, and practising relaxation and deep breathing. A feeling of drowsiness and lack of energy as well as poor sleep can also be helped by gentle physical activity, deep breathing and relaxation exercises. A persistently dry mouth can be helped by chewing sugarless chewing gum and drinking cold water or cold fruit juice. Withdrawal symptoms do not occur in everyone, and if they do occur in a moderate smoker of 15–20 cigarettes per day, they are unlikely to last longer than three weeks.

Gradual cessation of smoking—some useful steps

For heavy smokers, or for those who have smoked for many years, gradual withdrawal of smoking is often more useful than sudden and complete quitting. When using the method of gradually reducing your smoking habit, there are some steps which may help.

- If a non–filtered cigarette is smoked, *change to a filter tip cigarette*.
- Change to a cigarette which has a *lower nicotine content* than the one which is currently used.
- Gradually *reduce the number of cigarettes smoked each day*. The rate at which the number of cigarettes is reduced each day would be different for different individuals.
- When down to about ten cigarettes or less per day, *smoke only half of each cigarette, then only one-third of each cigarette*.
- *When ready to quit completely, certain other steps can help you.* Tell your family, friends and those at work that you are planning to quit, and ask for their help. Throw away all cigarette–connected articles such as ashtrays and cigarette lighters, not to mention cigarettes. Start to perform gentle

exercise, or if doing this already, slightly increase the exercise programme. Make the day of quitting smoking a special day, for example by going out to a nice restaurant for dinner or by buying oneself a gift.

- *Nicotine patch.* This can be useful for those who are heavy smokers and who appear to be addicted to the effects of nicotine. These individuals may get serious symptoms of withdrawal. This form of handling smoking cessation is simple, since a nicotine patch needs to be applied on the skin once per day for about three months. However, *it should be done under medical supervision*, and it is relatively expensive. It is also important to know that *smoking is dangerous whilst using a nicotine patch* because an abnormal rhythm of the heart can result when a person with a nicotine patch also smokes. Such an abnormal heartbeat is very occasionally a cause of death. Nicotine patch treatment has been found to work best in conjunction with counselling by a medical practitioner or a psychologist.

Other help during a quit smoking programme

There are a number of ways in which a person who is attempting to quit smoking can be helped. These will be described from the simplest to the most sophisticated, and clearly the last measures are best reserved for those who are heavily addicted to the tobacco habit or those who have quit and then relapsed.

Common-sense measures

- During the quitting programme, it is best to avoid friends who smoke and to avoid environments where smoking is prevalent, such as bars or nightclubs.
- Removal of all smoking-connected items such as ashtrays, cigarette lighters, the cleaning of motor vehicle ashtrays, and the cleaning of smoke-ridden clothes is all helpful.
- Alerting family, friends and those at the workplace that you are undertaking a quit programme is also very useful.
- It is also helpful if you can temporarily avoid being in

situations where you smoked previously, such as whilst watching television.

- Performing other activities when there is the urge to light up a cigarette are useful. These activities can include gentle physical activity such as walking or jogging, simple relaxation or deep breathing, and snacking on low-calorie foods such as pieces of fruit or raw vegetables, drinking water, mineral water or low-sugar fruit juice.

Anti-smoking support groups

It has been known for a long time that organised support groups consisting of ex-addicts can be important when dealing with any addictive behaviour associated with alcohol consumption, drug use or smoking. Organised support groups are a logical extension of the support probably already being provided by friends, family and those at work. The wonderful part of organised support groups is that they provide unconditional help, which is sometimes difficult in a family or work setting, and they can also provide special insights while sharing similar problems in relation to smoking cessation.

Professional counselling

Counselling by a medical practitioner or a behavioural expert such as a psychologist or counsellor, is most useful for someone who has been heavily addicted to tobacco use, for someone who is using a nicotine patch and for someone who has successfully quit smoking in the past and has relapsed again into the smoking habit.

While more expensive than the 'common-sense' measures described above, and that of organised support groups, professional counselling has the extra benefit of the wisdom and special experience of an expert. Sometimes a simple but strong request from an authority figure, such as one's medical practitioner, simply to 'stop smoking' can have an almost miraculous effect! Also, some special methods that are often employed by professional counsellors can be particularly useful for those who are prone to addictive behaviour and have a weak will.

Hypnotherapy

Hypnotherapy is best reserved for those in whom the other measures mentioned above have failed, and for whom it is really necessary to quit smoking for specific health reasons. During hypnotherapy, the individual undergoes a change in their state of consciousness in such a way that the hypnotherapist is able to suggest to the individual a change in their behaviour, in this case, to quit the smoking habit. It is essential to be sure that one is dealing with a certified hypnotherapist who has had experience in handling people who want to stop smoking.

What happens with a relapse?

This unfortunately occurs in about three out of four of those who have successfully but only temporarily been able to quit smoking. There can be many reasons for this, such as new life stresses, although often a relapse is due merely to the addictive nature of smoking. Eventually, most who relapse can quit smoking after a second, third or even fourth try. Essentially the same methods can be used as described above; however, the measures used during the quit programme usually need to become more structured and to involve additional methods, such as the use of a nicotine patch, support groups or professional counselling.

Is weight gain a problem during a quit smoking programme?

Many who stop smoking gain 2–3 kg (4–6 lbs) in weight. Probably the most important reason for this is a change in diet during the quitting process. Remember that it does no harm to gain 2–3 kg whilst undergoing the quit programme, and also that it is usually unwise and too difficult to also include a major dietary change during this time. However, during the quit programme one can do a few useful things by avoiding high-calorie food snacks such as biscuits, chocolate and other similar 'comfort' foods, and instead snack on low-calorie foods such as fruit, raw vegetables like carrots or celery, and eating plain popcorn and low calorie, low-fat biscuits, as well as by increasing the level of regular moderate physical activity.

Public health measures

> *We must not forget about public health measures which promote the overall idea that smoking is an unhealthy and socially unacceptable habit.*

The most important of these measures is education, and this education is best started in primary school in which the unhealthy nature of the tobacco habit is explained to the young brain, a brain which retains most information eagerly. It is also important to push politicians and public policy makers so that there are rules against smoking in public places, such as public buildings, restaurants, bars, nightclubs, airports and in aeroplanes. Politicians need to be pressured to legislate against the smoking habit, so that eventually we will live in a society which does not smoke, and in which the entire tobacco crop is replaced by other edible or otherwise usable crops.

7

Alcohol

> *Eat bread at pleasure,*
> *Drinke wine by measure.*
>
> *Randle Cosgrove (16th Century)*

Regular alcohol use is widespread in European and Western communities, as well as in some traditional cultures, and much myth, folklore, witty anecdote and romantic notions have surrounded its use.

> *Whilst a little alcohol may have some beneficial effects, the facts are that regular and excessive use of alcohol is harmful, causes several illnesses, including some cancers, and shortens the life of the heavy drinker by 10 to 15 years.*

ILL-HEALTH CAUSED BY ALCOHOL

The important hazards of regular and excessive alcohol consumption include failure of the liver to function normally. This is a serious problem because the liver can be considered to be the 'metabolic factory' or 'engine room' of the body. Brain cells are lost and brain function deteriorates over the years with excessive alcohol use. Alcohol is an important reason for loss of productivity, so that this habit influences the economy of the nation. Excessive alcohol consumption is an important cause of many motor vehicle accidents. Those who use alcohol excessively can be physically violent, and also display psychological violence within the family, and this can result in family breakup. Excessive alcohol consumption contributes to the development of some cancers which are shown in Table 7.1. It can be seen that excessive alcohol consumption is responsible for a wide range of illnesses, with sad and at times tragic family disruption, loss of productivity at work, and that the development of cancer is only one of its many ill-effects.

ALCOHOL AND CANCER

It has been estimated that in about 1 of every 20 cancers, alcohol consumption has been the main cause. Table 7.1 shows the cancers which regular alcohol consumption predisposes to.

Table 7.1: Alcohol-related cancers

Alcohol a proven cause	Alcohol a likely contributory cause
Mouth cancer	Colon cancer
Throat cancer	Rectal cancer
Gullet (oesophagus) cancer	Colon adenomas (polyps)
Primary liver cancer	Rectal adenomas (polyps)
	Breast cancer

How much is too much alcohol?

Drink not the third glasse
Which thou canst tame
When once it is within thee

George Herbert (1593–1633)

Alcohol consumption is generally measured in units, each of which contains about 10–12 g of alcohol. This amounts to one nip of spirits, one glass of wine, or an average glass of beer. While these measures are approximate only, they allow us to compare different alcoholic drinks.

Recent scientific studies have linked alcohol consumption in moderation, 1–2 drinks per day, with prolongation of life and a degree of protection from several illnesses, in particular from heart disease and narrowing of the arteries in both men and women, when compared to non-users of alcohol. Some would say that any amount of alcohol is harmful, but the scientific evidence contradicts this view.

At least in the development of a cancer such as colon cancer or rectal cancer, three or more daily drinks of alcohol consumed for 20 years or longer, can be a contributory cause of these cancers in men, while this amount is probably less for women. Scientists believe that in a cancer prevention programme it is unwise to drink more than three standard alcoholic drinks per day for a man and two for a woman. It is known that five or six alcoholic drinks each day markedly increases the risk of developing alcohol-related cancers and other medical conditions associated with alcohol use, and that ten or more standard drinks per day would almost guarantee that the individual will develop an alcohol-related illness which will markedly shorten the life of the drinker.

Is it the type of alcohol which is consumed, or is it the amount of alcohol which is the important cause in the development of cancer? It seems that the amount of alcohol consumed is the most important factor. However, studies in relation to colon and rectal cancer, and the precancerous colo-rectal adenomas, suggest that over and above the amount of alcohol consumed, there is something in beer, but not in wine, which is an additional risk for these tumours.

How alcohol contributes to cancer

Whilst scientists are undecided whether alcohol causes cancer directly or indirectly, or in both ways, this is really not important for the person at risk, as the end result is that regular and excessive alcohol consumption is known to predispose to several cancers. Alcohol probably exerts its effect as a cancer-producing agent in one of several ways.

- *Damages the cells of the body, such as liver cells or the lining cells of the gut.* This can result in an abnormally rapid turnover of cells, a factor in the development of cancer.
- *Contains or produces carcinogens.* Substances such as nitrosamines and urethane are found or produced in the body as a result of drinking some alcoholic beverages such as beer, whisky, bourbon and brandy.
- *Suppresses the immune system.* Heavy alcohol consumption suppresses the immune response and diminishes its capacity to defend itself against cancer cells, which when few in number are usually effectively disposed of by the normal immune system of the body.
- *Causes nutritional deficiencies.* For example, it depletes the body of important vitamins such as folic acid, vitamin C and beta-carotene, and trace minerals such as selenium, nutrients which normally can assist in cancer prevention.
- *Alters the function of enzymes.* Alcohol can deactivate some enzymes which can repair damaged DNA, and it can also activate some other enzymes which change an inert substance in the body into a carcinogen.
- *Alters hormone levels.* Alcohol increases oestrogen levels, and this may be a factor in the known increased breast cancer risk among those women who consume excessive alcohol.

HOW TO HANDLE ALCOHOL AS PART OF CANCER PREVENTION

If you are a daily alcohol consumer now, *have at least two alcohol-free days every week.* During these alcohol-free days substitute water, mineral water, tonic water, tomato juice with lemon and spices (a 'Virgin Mary') for alcoholic beverages, or some non-alcohol containing beer or wine which has the taste but not the alcohol content. 'Binge drinking' should be avoided.

On the days when alcohol is drunk, try some low alcohol content drinks, such as low alcohol beer, low alcohol wine, or a wine spritzer, which is a mixture of wine and mineral or soda water.

Regular alcohol consumers should eat well, and particularly eat plenty of vegetables, fruit, grains, cereals and fish (Chapter 5). These foods contain a lot of vitamin C, folic acid, and selenium, substances which are known to counteract the ill-effects of alcohol consumption in relation to the development of cancer.

If alcohol consumption is a life problem, it may be necessary to stop drinking alcohol completely by changing to non-alcoholic drinks, non-alcohol beer and wine, by commencing a gentle exercise programme and taking part in relaxation and meditation regularly. If these simple measures are not successful, then it may become necessary to turn to Alcoholics Anonymous or other similar organisations, or seek professional help in order to quit the alcohol habit.

If a person drinks alcohol twice or more often each week, it is wise to limit it to no more than three alcoholic drinks per day for a man and to no more than two alcoholic drinks per day for a woman.

8

Sun

At twelve noon,
The natives swoon,
And no further work is done,
But mad dogs and Englishmen
Go out in the midday sun.

Sir Nöel Coward (1899–1973)

The sun is essential to the survival of our planet, and the energy derived from it allows plants to grow. Daylight and sunlight give us a feeling of well-being and vitality. Also, our bodies are able to manufacture vitamin D as a result of ultraviolet radiation emanating from the sun.

Unfortunately, excessive exposure to the sun's rays damages the skin. This is the single most important cause of both malignant melanomas and non-melanoma skin cancers. Radiation damage from the sun is responsible for about 2% of all cancer deaths in developed countries.

Malignant melanomas can be fatal. Every year about 40,000 people are diagnosed in the USA, and in a small country such as Australia with only 18 million people, about 6000 individuals develop this cancer each year.

Non-melanoma skin cancers are much more common than malignant melanomas, and while they are usually not fatal, they can cause a great deal of disability and disfigurement, and add many millions each year to the national health bill. These non-melanoma skin cancers are of two types, *basal cell carcinoma* and *squamous cell carcinoma*. The causes and prevention of these skin cancers are discussed in more detail in Chapter 18. Here, a general picture is presented of the ill-effects of excessive sunlight, and the ways in which you can control this.

WHY EXCESSIVE SUNLIGHT IS HARMFUL

The energy of sunlight (solar radiation) consists of a mixture of ultraviolet rays of varying wavelengths, UVA being the longest wavelength, UVB the medium wavelength, and UVC the shortest wavelength. Ozone in the upper atmosphere absorbs most of these ultraviolet rays and only a small amount of UVA and UVB reaches the earth. UVB radiation burns the skin and is probably the most important cancer-producing agent. In recent years experimental studies in animals have suggested that UVA rays which do not usually burn the skin but penetrate the skin layer more deeply, may also be a cancer-producing agent, but this has so far not been confirmed in humans.

Nobody's skin is immune from damage by excessive sunlight. However, individuals with certain types of skin, such as those with pale skin, those who have many freckles, blue or light-coloured eyes, red or fair hair, who develop sunburn easily and often tan with difficulty, are more prone to skin damage and skin cancers than are those with olive or dark skin. Excessive sunlight is therefore a relative term, and largely depends on the type of skin an individual possesses. However, it is important to know that any type of skin can be damaged by sunlight.

The top layer of our skin is shed constantly, and this means that at the bottom layer of the skin, cells are constantly dividing. Over a period of time a precancerous condition emerges when these dividing cells are damaged by sunlight, producing a genetic change in the dividing cells, which is then reproduced in the next cell division. This precancerous condition is usually just a small circumscribed roughened area of the exposed skin. With the passage of time, and with further damage by the sun, further genetic changes occur in the dividing cells, and the eventual result is a skin cancer.

This progression from a normal cell to a precancerous cell, and then to an actual cancer cell, takes some years, and it is related to the total amount of ultraviolet radiation received on the skin, and also on the number of episodes of sunburn, particularly if that sunburn occurs in adolescence and young adulthood.

WHO IS AT RISK OF SKIN DAMAGE BY SUNLIGHT?

This can be answered by three main considerations, which to some extent overlap.

- *Those who have inherited a fair complexion* with pale skin, blue or light-coloured eyes, many freckles, often many moles, red or fair hair, who have difficulty tanning and whose skin burns rapidly when exposed to sunlight. However, if you are olive-skinned or dark-skinned, don't think that you are immune from damage by excessive ultraviolet rays.
- *Those who during their life have received large quantities of ultraviolet radiation* from the sun or from tanning machines.
- *Those who have had one or more episodes of severe sunburn*, and particularly if these episodes occurred during childhood, adolescence or young adult life.

Limiting the Damaging Effects of Excessive Sunlight

Public education has been very effective in countries such as Australia, letting the community know that excessive exposure to sunlight can be prevented by simple measures. Commencing this education at primary school would make an enormous difference to the many skin cancers which are currently found in developed countries such as the USA, UK and Australia. The primary and secondary prevention of skin cancers is discussed in great detail in Chapter 18, and here I merely suggest briefly that there are three measures which will minimise skin damage and will greatly lower skin cancer rates.

- *Limit exposure to the sun*, especially when the sun's rays are overhead, and therefore at their most penetrating. This occurs between 10 in the morning and 3 in the afternoon. Also stay in the shade whenever possible, especially for those who have a fair complexion.
- *Cover up the exposed parts of the body.* Wear a hat, long-sleeved shirt or blouse, and trousers or slacks.
- *Use suitable sunscreen* on those parts of the body which cannot be covered up, or during physical activity in which sports clothes need to be worn that expose the limbs, such as when swimming, playing tennis or cycling.

In Chapter 18, where the causes and prevention of skin cancers are discussed in detail, it can be seen that the benefits of sunlight and sunshine can still be obtained and that sunlight skin damage can be minimised, thereby removing from our lives many skin cancers.

9

Physical activity

Those who think they have not time for bodily exercise
will sooner or later have to find time for illness.

Edward Stanley, the Earl of Derby
(1826–1893)

We know that humans at the end of the Stone Age engaged in extensive physical activity, that they had a wonderful diet even by modern standards, and experienced little cancer. In 1912, a member of the English aristocracy, the Honourable Rollo Russell, who had no formal scientific training, but who collected a lot of information about the causes and prevention of cancer in a book he wrote that year called *Preventable Cancer*, among other thought-provoking statements, declared that 'sedentary occupations are highly injurious for cancer'.

It will come as no surprise that regular, moderate physical activity affords protection against several illnesses, and forms part of a sound lifestyle. In the past fifteen years scientists have also researched a possible relationship between various forms of cancer and physical activity. The cancers which have been most studied in this regard are cancers of the colon and rectum, adenomatous polyps of the colon and rectum, and to a lesser extent, cancers of the breast, uterus, ovary, prostate and testicle (Table 9.1). It was first observed in the early 1980s that men with sedentary occupations were prone to cancer of the colon and it was from this observation that further research was undertaken to test the role of physical activity in relation to the causes of various cancers.

Table 9.1: Physical inactivity and cancer risk

Colon cancer
Colon adenoma
Breast cancer
Testicular cancer
Ovarian cancer
Prostate cancer
Uterine cancer

HOW PHYSICAL ACTIVITY INFLUENCES CANCER RISK

There are probably several ways in which physical activity might decrease the risk of certain cancers.

- *Decrease of body fat.* Excessive fat is a risk factor for all the cancers which appear in Table 9.1, with the exception of testicular cancer. Regular physical activity influences body weight and body fat. Moreover, female hormones, which are related to cancers of the breast, uterus and ovary, are in part stored in fat, so if less fat is present, less of these hormones are available to be released.
- *Stimulates immune function.* Research shows that moderate exercise stimulates and improves the immune function of the body. This means that the body can better defend itself against illness and can better deal with any cancer cells which may be present in the body. However, extreme physical activity, such as running a marathon, depletes the

immune system, and extreme and exhausting physical activity should be avoided in any cancer prevention programme.

- *Hormonal changes.* Moderate regular exercise favourably alters the hormonal balance in women, thereby producing a protective effect for cancers of the breast, uterus and ovary. It is possible that in men testosterone levels are lowered with moderate physical activity, and this may contribute to protection against cancer of the prostate.
- *Large bowel transit.* In many individuals, moderate physical activity increases the speed with which large bowel contents are moved towards the rectum for evacuation. This increased rate of bowel transit is a possible, though so far unproven reason for the demonstrated protective effect of physical activity for colon cancer and the precancerous colon adenoma.

How to exercise

The sovereign invigorator of the body is exercise.
Not less than two hours a day should be devoted to exercise.

Thomas Jefferson (1743–1826)

Perhaps taking their lead from President Thomas Jefferson, scientists in the USA have been the most prominent in recent years in determining the optimum level of exercise that is useful for the maintenance of good health and for the prevention of illness, including cancer.

At least 30 minutes of moderate exercise, in which the heart rate (pulse rate) is raised, or in which one sweats a little, performed at least five days of each week is recommended for the maintenance of good health and for the prevention of illness. *In the presence of heart or lung disease, or some other chronic illness, such as arthritis, or if there is a concern that this physical activity may in fact be harmful, it is essential to consult a medical practitioner before embarking on an exercise programme.*

For those who at present are not doing physical activity regularly, the type of exercise which can be performed in most climates year round, and which does not involve excessive cost, includes brisk walking, jogging or running (these last two produce wear and tear on joints and ligaments), swimming, cycling and gymnasium work. Apart from regular and planned physical activity along the lines described above, think physical, and fit physical activity into your daily life, for example by walking briskly or jogging to neighbourhood stores, walking up and down stairs instead of using elevators, and whenever possible, walking or cycling instead of using a motor vehicle.

Thirty minutes or more of moderate physical activity, which raises the pulse or makes one sweat a little, five days or more often each week, such as brisk walking, jogging, cycling, swimming or doing gymnasium work, will not only be a help towards maintaining good health and be a protection from various illnesses, including several cancers, but will also add a sense of vitality and well-being to life.

10

Sexual activity

The sexual revolution is over and the microbes won.

Give War a Chance
Patrick J. O'Rourke (1947–)

Although some say that good sex makes the world go round, the downside of this is that some viruses can be passed between individuals during sexual intercourse, in the fluids of the semen and vagina, and from other parts of the genitalia. The problem is that some of these viruses predispose the person so infected to certain cancers. One in six of the world's cancer deaths have been attributed to viruses, and most of these deaths occur in developing countries. The viruses involved and the type of cancer resulting from such an infection are summarised in Table 10.1.

- *Human papilloma virus (HPV)* is transmitted by sexual inter-course and eventually forms visible wart-like outgrowths around the vagina, cervix, penis and the anus, the last usually in those who practise anal intercourse. This virus appears to be a most important precancerous condition in cancer of

Table 10.1: Sexually transmitted viruses predisposing to cancer

Virus involved	Type of cancer
Human papilloma virus (HPV) Herpes simplex II (genital herpes)	Cervix cancer Vaginal cancer Penis cancer Anal cancer
Human immunodeficiency virus (HIV)—progresses to acquired immunodeficiency syndrome (AIDS)	Lymphoma Kaposi sarcoma
Hepatitis B virus Hepatitis C virus (uncommonly sexually transmitted)	Liver cancer

the cervix, and it also predisposes to cancer of the penis, anal cancer, and vaginal cancer.

- *Herpes simplex II* or *genital herpes virus* also appears to predispose individuals to cervix cancer as well as to penis and anal cancer, although the evidence for this association is less well established than for the human papilloma virus.

- *Human immunodeficiency virus (HIV)* progresses in most individuals to what is almost always the fatal condition of the *acquired immunodeficiency syndrome* (AIDS). This virus causes a dramatic depression of the human immune system, and among other serious illnesses, predisposes the individual to malignant lymphomas, which are malignant tumours of the lymph glands. Another malignant tumour associated with HIV and AIDS is *Kaposi sarcoma*, named after the skin specialist Dr Moritz Kaposi, who first described this condition, well before HIV and AIDS were even heard of. This malignant tumour usually makes its appearance first as pigmented nodules in the skin, but it can spread subsequently to the rest of the body.

- *Hepatitis B virus* is probably the most common sexually transmitted virus. This virus can be transmitted in other ways apart from sexual intercourse. It is usually transmitted by 'carriers' of the virus. These carriers are usually in good health and appear to have recovered completely from their hepatitis B infection. A small proportion of individuals who develop hepatitis B do not clear the virus from their bodies, and remain as virus carriers and can transmit this virus to other individuals by sexual intercourse, and also in the saliva. Hepatitis B infection predisposes an individual to the development of primary liver cancer. Hepatitis B infection can be effectively prevented by immunisation.

- *Hepatitis C virus* has been discovered more recently and can also cause liver cancer. This complication has been frequent in some countries, such as Japan. Hepatitis C is mainly transmitted through blood transfusion, if the blood has not been screened for hepatitis C, and also through infected syringes and needles in intravenous drug users, and during body piercing and tattooing using unclean instruments. Sexual intercourse is a possible but uncommon means of transmitting hepatitis C.

SEXUAL PRACTICE IN A CANCER PREVENTION PROGRAMME

The prevention of sexually transmitted disease is outside the scope of this book, and here I merely describe briefly those aspects which we need to be concerned with when advising on a comprehensive cancer prevention programme. The approach to sexual practice in relation to cancer prevention depends very much on whether the sexual relationship is with only one heterosexual partner, or whether there are multiple sex partners, whether there is anal intercourse, or whether there is a bisexual relationship.

- *Single heterosexual partner.* In such a stable relationship, the sexual history of the two partners can almost always be freely discussed, and if neither partner has a history or a possibility of a past sexually transmitted disease such as genital herpes, genital warts or papillomas, or hepatitis B, then no particular protective measures are necessary. If there is any doubt, then it is useful to have blood tests for HIV and hepatitis B carrier status. If these tests are negative, no special precautions are necessary in relation to virus transmission during sexual intercourse. If the tests are positive, then the male partner should be advised to use a condom.

- *Multiple partners or anal intercourse.* A condom should be used during intercourse. Anyone in this situation who develops a lump, ulcer, swelling or a wart around the vagina, penis or anus, needs to have this checked immediately by a medical practitioner. Women who are at high risk for developing cancer of the cervix because of their sexual history, that is, many partners, sexual intercourse started soon after puberty, or a history of a genital wart or ulcer, need to have regular screening tests as described in Chapter 19, which deals with cancer of the cervix.

Reducing the risk of sexually transmitted viruses is possible by appropriate preventive action. This is usually relatively simple, and can diminish the chances of developing many serious illnesses, including cancer. Remember that HIV and AIDS, a disease which is almost always fatal, can usually also be prevented.

11

Stress

Cases are so frequent in which deep anxiety, deferred hope and disappointment are quickly followed by the growth and increase of cancer.

Surgical Pathology
Sir James Paget (1814–1899)

When we are challenged by stressful changes in life, such as the loss of one's spouse, our resistance to disease can be lowered, and as a result we can become ill with all types of illnesses, including cancer. This of course does not mean that every major stressful event in life is followed by an illness of some type, but it does mean that if there are several such events, the chances of developing an illness, to which one is probably also otherwise predisposed for reasons other than stress, is higher than if such events did not take place.

We now have a respectable body of scientific evidence which shows a relationship between major stresses in life and the development of various cancers. Scientists have also been able to tell us how such changes may lead to various forms of illness, including cancer.

CAN STRESSFUL EVENTS RESULT IN ILLNESS?

The short answer to this question is 'yes, but not always'. The long answer is that there needs to be a certain set of circumstances present before stressful life events can trigger an illness, including cancer. There needs to be a perception by the individual that these events are stressful and negative, that the individual has difficulty coping with the situation, and that those individuals who develop a particular illness are also predisposed to that illness for other reasons, such as an inherited susceptibility or some lifestyle problem such as a poor diet or smoking.

It seems that stressful events in life can be a 'trigger' for the appearance of an illness, and that other factors must also be present before that illness occurs. This probably means that stress does not usually cause an illness on its own, and also that the stressful changes in life are present reasonably close to the appearance of the illness. With cancer, it has been found that these stressful events need to be present for about 5–10 years before the cancer is diagnosed. Stressful events which occurred 15, 20 or 30 years before the cancer was diagnosed do not seem to be important, but more recent events over the previous few years can be important.

So what is this combination of factors in relation to life stress which increases a person's chance of developing an illness, including cancer?

- *Number and type of stressful events.* Two American scientists, Dr Thomas Holmes and Dr Richard Rahe, have researched the importance of different stressful life changes and have given each a rating. For example, death of a spouse rates 100 points, retirement rates 45 points, sexual difficulties rate 39 points, and so on. They could predict a serious illness developing in a person who in one year has accumulated a rating of over 300 points.
- *Life change causing prolonged upset (inability to adjust or cope).* Several scientists have found that if a person remains upset for an unduly long time, such as being upset for years and

years after bereavement, then they have a higher chance of developing an illness, including cancer, than those who can adjust within a reasonable period of time. This was well expressed by William Shakespeare, who in *Hamlet* had one of his actors say, 'There is nothing either good or bad, but thinking makes it so'.

- *There is a hereditary or lifestyle predisposition also.* It seems that stressful life changes, and a prolonged period of upsetness because of these life changes, are by themselves not sufficient for an illness to develop. In most cases there also needs to be some predisposition to it, such as a poor diet, smoking, alcohol abuse, or an inherited predisposition. This means that we need to look on stressful life changes not as a direct cause of illness, but rather as a trigger which brings the condition to the attention of the individual. With cancer, it is believed that a few cancer cells are already present for reasons such as poor diet, smoking, alcohol abuse or inherited factors. The addition of stressful life changes then lowers the individual's resistance and ability to deal with and remove in the usual way these few cancer cells that are present in the body. As a consequence, these cells are allowed to multiply and produce symptoms. It is then that the person attends a medical practitioner and the cancer is diagnosed.

- *Stress changes life habits.* Don't forget that stressful events in life can also alter our behaviour. For example, as a consequence of stressful events, we might begin to smoke excessively or drink alcohol excessively, or eat the wrong foods, and these changes in habits, if they are continued, can themselves contribute to the causation of a cancer.

So stress is a complicated issue, not completely understood, nor entirely explicable by scientists. Nevertheless, it seems that in many instances, stressful events can trigger an illness, including cancer. For cancer, the stressful events need to be present a few years before the actual cancer is diagnosed.

CANCERS THAT MAY BE STRESS RELATED

At present the evidence is suggestive, but it is certainly not proven scientifically that stressful events may be a contributory cause of cancer. The strongest evidence that stressful life changes can trigger certain cancers is for cancer of the colon, cancer of the rectum, breast cancer and lung cancer. However, it is very unlikely that this triggering effect of stress is only present for these cancers. The more likely explanation is that all cancers can be triggered by stressful life changes and by the emotional change which is often associated with these stresses, and that these four cancers have shown up mainly because they are common cancers and therefore have been more extensively studied by scientists than the less common malignant tumours.

HOW STRESS MIGHT TRIGGER CANCER

Scientists are still piecing the clues together, and at present the explanations of how stress may be a triggering factor in the appearance of a cancer should be regarded as speculative. Extensive studies in certain well-defined groups of individuals who are known to be under major stresses, such as among those who have had a bereavement and who do not adjust and remain in grief for an abnormally long period of time, have shown that their immunity often becomes depressed, so that they are more susceptible to various illnesses, including cancer. This lowering of the immunity interferes with the normal capacity of the body to eliminate the occasional cancer cell which may be present in the body. This depression of the immune state allows the multiplication of these cells, and as a result a lump appears, say in the breast, which is then diagnosed as breast cancer.

STRESS MANAGEMENT IN A CANCER PREVENTION PROGRAMME

At present scientists cannot say with certainty that reducing one's stress level will decrease the risk of developing a cancer. The evidence for this is mounting, suggesting that stress can be a trigger for the appearance of a cancer, but the evidence is not nearly as strong as say for diet, smoking and inherited factors. Nevertheless, I present some methods which may be useful in reducing your stress level, in the knowledge that if performed correctly, they can do you no harm, your life is likely to become more vital and enjoyable, and as a bonus, your chances of developing a cancer or other illnesses may also be reduced.

Given that avoiding stressful situations cannot often be achieved, we turn to the many ways in which we can reduce our stress level. In the incomplete state of our knowledge, I would certainly not advocate complex techniques of stress reduction, such as biofeedback and hypnotherapy, methods which are best reserved for those individuals who are highly stressed and unable to conduct their daily life because of it. I would like to briefly mention the value of exercise, of life enjoyment, relaxation, meditation, yoga and imagery techniques, as well as the technique of autogenic training.

Exercise

Physical activity provides a sense of well-being to the individual, and has been known to be an important stress reduction technique for many years. It is now known that immunity is boosted by gentle or moderate exercise. Moreover, compounds called *endorphins* are released during physical activity, and these are similar to morphine, producing a natural form of elation, without the use of drugs. It was suggested in Chapter 9 that 30 minutes or more of physical activity which raises the pulse and causes some sweating, performed five or more days per week, will do it. Brisk walking, jogging, running, cycling, swimming or gymnasium work are all simple and useful methods. *If there are concerns about embarking on a programme of physical activity for health reasons, please consult a medical practitioner first.*

Life enjoyment

For hundreds of years wise doctors have held that if we are able to enjoy our life, our work, our family, our friends, have interests and hobbies and do regular physical activity, then we will not be stressed. This of course is sometimes difficult to put into practice, but we should strive for this in our daily lives.

Relaxation, meditation, imagery

Relaxation exercises and the use of meditation take relatively little time, and are a wonderful means of reducing one's stress level. There are many books and audio tapes as well as relaxation and meditation classes which one can attend to learn these techniques. Imagery is an activity in which one is instructed to recall beautiful places and other pleasurable images as a means of stress reduction. These techniques are often recommended for cancer patients. However, they can be equally well used by anyone wishing to reduce their stress levels. It is important to be taught imagery properly by appropriate experts.

Autogenic training

This is a technique in which one is taught to give some simple commands when in a relaxed state, such as when lying on a sofa, and in which various parts of the body become relaxed, thereby reducing the overall level of stress. This method was developed in Germany well before the Second World War and has surfaced again as one of the 'New Age' techniques. Again, it is important that the technique of autogenic training is taught by an expert.

We of course don't know for sure whether successful stress management would help to prevent cancer. The scientific evidence is mounting that it may at least remove one of the triggers which allows a cancer in a predisposed individual to grow and spread. It is certain though that there are no side-effects from properly taught stress reduction techniques, and that successful reduction of stress levels is very likely to provide more vitality and enjoyment of life, something we can all benefit from in this complex and often stressful life which most of us lead.

12

The workplace

There is a disease as peculiar to a certain set of people,
which has not, at least to my knowledge, been
publickly noticed, I mean the chimney sweepers' cancer.
The disease is brought on them by their occupation.
The disease in these people, seems to derive its origin
from a lodgement of soot in the rugae of the scrotum.

The Chirurgical Works of Percivall Pott, FRS
Percivall Pott (1714–1788)

Writing thus about cancer of the scrotum in chimney sweeps, the noted 18th century English surgeon, Mr Percivall Pott, unwittingly opened the door on what we now call *occupational cancer*. One in every 25 cancers has been mainly contributed to by occupational causes. Fortunately, strict control measures in the workplace enforced over the past generation have halved, at least in developed countries, the number of workplace-related cancers. The number of occupations in which there is an elevated risk for cancer is extensive, and there is a long list of likely or known cancer-producing agents in the workplace. It is possible that work-related stresses can trigger the development of a malignant tumour in someone who is susceptible to it.

However, scientific knowledge of this link is in its infancy, and whilst we are likely to learn much more about this in the future, at present one cannot make any specific recommendations except to reduce one's stress levels at work, just as one does in out-of-work life by using the simple methods described earlier in Chapter 11.

OCCUPATION AND CANCER RISK

Table 12.1 is a selection of occupations, listed in alphabetical order. It provides an indication of the particular chemical or physical agent which is thought to be the carcinogen responsible, together with the actual cancer to which workers in the occupation group are susceptible. This list is a partial reference for some of the common and important occupations in which there is an increased chance of developing cancer. If there is any doubt about a particular occupation being a cancer risk, please consult an occupational health physician or the occupational health consultant or agency at the workplace, the union, the environmental protection authority, or some other similar agency.

Table 12.1: Occupation and cancer risk

Occupation	Likely carcinogenic agent	Site of cancer risk
Asbestos worker (mining, shipyards, insulation, rubber tyres, demolition, brake-lining)	Asbestos fibre	Lung Mesothelioma Throat
Brick and ceramic manufacture	Arsenic Beryllium Chromium	Skin Lung Nose Throat Liver
Cadmium production (metal workers, electroplating, nuclear plants)	Cadmium	Lung Prostate

Table 12.1: Occupation and cancer risk (cont.)

Occupation	Likely carcinogenic agent	Site of cancer risk
Chemical workers	Aminobiphenyl Benzene Benzidine Chloromethyl ether Cadmium Chromium 2-Naphthylamine	Leukaemia Pancreas Bladder Lung Prostate Throat
Chromium and alloy production	Chromium and chromium compounds	Lung Nose Throat
Coal/gas, shale-oil production, coke plant workers	Aromatic hydrocarbons Coke-oven gases and vapours	Lung Skin Bladder Pancreas
Copper production (smelters, electrolysis)	2-naphthylamine	Bladder Pancreas
Dye workers	Aminobiphenyl Benzidine 2-naphthylamine	Bladder Pancreas
Electrical/electronic workers (electricians, radio/TV repairers, telephone and computer mechanics)	Electromagnetic fields (EMF) Beryllium	Leukaemia Lymphoma Brain Bladder
Electroplaters/electrolysis workers	Cadmium 2-naphthylamine	Lung Prostate Bladder Pancreas
Farmers and agricultural workers	Ultraviolet radiation Pesticides/weed killers	Skin Lip Lymphoma Leukaemia Prostate Lung Soft tissue sarcoma
Garage and transport workers	Diesel exhaust	Lung
Glass manufacture	Arsenic Chromium compounds	Skin Lung Liver Nose Throat
Hairdressers	Hair dyes	Bladder
Insulation workers	Asbestos fibre	Lung Mesothelioma Throat

Table 12.1: Occupation and cancer risk (cont.)

Occupation	Likely carcinogenic agent	Site of cancer risk
Leather and shoe workers	Benzene	Leukaemia
	Isopropyl	Sinuses
Nickel production	Nickel	Lung
	2-naphthylamine	Nose
		Bladder
		Pancreas
Nuclear plant/nuclear power workers	Beryllium	Bladder
	Cadmium	Lung
		Prostate
Painters	Painting material	Lung
	Benzene	Leukaemia
Office workers	Tobacco smoke	Lung
		Throat
Petroleum workers	Arsenic	Skin
	Benzene	Lung
	Petroleum	Leukaemia
		Gallbladder and bile duct
Plastics workers	Vinyl chloride	Liver
		Lymphoma
		Lung
Radiologists, radiographers	Ionizing radiation	Skin
		Thyroid
		Brain
		Lung
		Breast
		Bone
		Pancreas
		Leukaemia
		Myeloma
Rubber, rubber tyre manufacture	Asbestos fibre	Lung
	Benzene	mesothelioma
	Auramine	Leukaemia
	2-naphthylamine	Bladder
		Pancreas
		gallbladder and bile duct
Shipyard workers	Asbestos fibre	Lung
		Mesothelioma
		Throat
Steel workers	Coke-oven gases and vapours	Lung
		Kidney
Tanners	Arsenic	Skin
		Lung

Table 12.1: Occupation and cancer risk (cont.)

Occupation	Likely carcinogenic agent	Site of cancer risk
Uranium miners	Ionizing radiation Radon gas	Skin Thyroid Brain Lung Breast Bone Pancreas Leukaemia Myeloma
Waiters/bartenders	Tobacco smoke	Lung Throat
Woodworkers (carpenters, furniture makers, polishers and finishers)	Wood dust Benzene	Nose Sinuses Throat Leukaemia

A CANCER PREVENTION PROGRAMME AT THE WORKPLACE

In most developed countries there are legislative and regulatory measures, in keeping with what is known about health hazards at work, including the hazards of developing a malignant tumour. In most countries also, apart from the regulatory bodies, there are accident and ill-health prevention departments in large places of employment, including a health and safety officer, and there are often departments which deal with health and safety at the workplace in unions. Moreover, there exist also environmental protection authorities and other similar bodies with accessible and usually free provision of information, and there are also occupational health physicians who are experts in the means of prevention and risk minimisation of illnesses, including workplace-related cancers.

The following are some general guidelines and principles for minimising your risk of developing cancer at the workplace.

- *Educate yourself about potential cancer hazards in the workplace.* Some workplaces do not present any additional hazards in relation to developing a malignant tumour.

- *Wear protective gear* if dealing with substances which are suspected or known to promote a particular cancer. This may include protective clothing, gloves, shoes, hats, masks and respirators. If there is a chance of contamination of the gear, don't take it home. Clean all gear meticulously, using the recommended methods. If chemicals are spilled, change clothes, wash clothes and do whatever is appropriate for that particular substance.

- *Advise your employer if protection is insufficient.* If there is a suspicion that the workplace takes inadequate precautions to protect workers from a cancer risk, then it is necessary to bring this to the attention of the employer or union representative, or both. These are difficult times industrially and economically in the Western world, and those who involve the employer in this way need to do so in a sensible, rational and non-confrontational manner in the first instance. It is often helpful to point out to the employer that some of these hazards, for example tobacco smoke in the work environment, are an additional cost to the employer in terms of productivity. The costs flow from the number of days which may be missed at work as a result of the health effects of the smoke, as well as from the economic disadvantages for the employer and for the community.

In approaching the 21st century we have considerable information on effective ways of minimising cancer risk in the workplace. There is no good reason why these protective measures, which are usually quite simple, should not be adhered to, so that the worker can enjoy the work environment, and increase productivity without the fear of developing ill-health, including work-related cancer.

13

Home and environment

For a man's house is his castle,
and the safest refuge to everyone.

Sir Edward Coke (1552–1634)

The home, garden, and out-of-work environment are usually wonderful for our health and well-being, and only infrequently contribute to the development of a cancer. Environmental pollution is a very uncommon cause of cancer, and air pollution is usually also a negligible factor. Very high levels of air pollution, particularly from diesel exhaust, may slightly increase the risk of lung cancer. The drinking water in developed countries is usually safe, and there are effective systems in operation to test for major contaminants in municipal water systems. Radon gas, to be described shortly, can occasionally seep from the soil into wells. Radon gas can be a hazard if the water supply comes from a well which has not been tested. Fortunately, not many people live close to nuclear plants or chemical waste dump areas. Moreover, not only is the home and surrounding environment relatively safe in most situations, if there is any doubt, some fairly simple measures can be taken to detect and eliminate environmental cancer hazards, thereby further reducing the risk of cancer.

Table 13.1 lists six potential household and environmental cancer hazards, and these, put together, probably form the main risks for cancer in the home and environment in developed countries.

Table 13.1: Some household and environmental cancer hazards

- Tobacco smoke—passive smoking
- Asbestos fibre
- Radon gas
- Pesticides
- Household cleaners, solvents and chemicals
- Electromagnetic fields (EMF)

TOBACCO SMOKE—PASSIVE SMOKING

Although the unhealthy effects of another person's tobacco smoke are being increasingly recognised, it needs to be stated again that passive smoking still remains responsible for several instances of lung cancer, and a few instances of throat cancer. Moreover, passive or second-hand smoke can cause chest infections and asthma, especially in children, and may also be in part responsible for some cases of the sudden infant death syndrome (SIDS).

It's wonderful to note an increasing volume of legislation which prohibits smoking in public places, as well as an increasing number of rules in offices, factories and in the workplace in general which prohibit smoking.

It is now the duty and responsibility of those in a household to insist that if anyone smokes, they do it outdoors.

110

ASBESTOS FIBRE

Asbestos is an excellent building and insulating material which has been used in homes during the 20th century, for roofing, pipe insulation and as part of floor tiles. Unfortunately, asbestos fibres crumble easily, and small particles which can be seen only under the microscope, get into the air, and can stick to one's body and clothing. When inhaled or swallowed, they can lodge in the throat and lungs and sometimes go down the gut, into the stomach and bowel, and can cause damage which sometimes leads to cancer. Most importantly, it can cause cancer of the lung and of the lining of the lung (*mesothelioma*), the throat (larynx), and possibly also cancers of the gullet, stomach, colon and ovary.

Asbestos fibre is only dangerous when it becomes damaged. Should asbestos in poor or damaged condition be suspected, contact the environmental protection authority or some similar organisation for further information. They can also advise about means of identifying whether there is a risk, and if so, the best way to remove the asbestos hazard.

An asbestos fibre problem can be suspected, particularly in an older home (built between 1930 and 1960), in which hot water systems or woodstoves or other similar equipment were insulated with material containing asbestos fibre. Other potential sources of asbestos fibre are vinyl floors in which there is asbestos, also roofing and siding shingles containing asbestos, and sometimes sound proofing or decorative painting, which in the past has been sprayed onto the walls of houses.

It is most unwise for an untrained individual to try to deal with any potential asbestos fibre problem in the home. If there is asbestos fibre danger at home, it is essential to obtain the help of experts who are certified by the relevant environmental protection authority, or other similar agencies, to advise on any asbestos removal and clean up which may be necessary.

RADON GAS

Radon gas is the breakdown product of uranium. It is radio-active, can be present in the soil or in rock, and can be a cause of lung cancer. This gas can come into a house, usually from below, through gaps and cracks in the floor and walls, or through gaps around pipes or cement construction joints. It is sometimes also present in the water supply if water comes from wells. It is more common to find higher radon levels in countries which frequently build houses with basements, such as in the USA and Europe, than it is in countries such as Australia where basements are uncommon and where houses are not hermetically sealed from below, and therefore have plenty of ventilation.

Testing for radon gas

There are both short-term devices in which radon testing can be done over a period of two to three days, or longer term testing which may take three months to assess the amount of radon in the home. This equipment can usually be obtained from both private contractors or public utilities, and is usually relatively inexpensive.

Lowering household radon levels

If radon testing suggests an abnormal elevation of radon in the house, it is best to contact the local environmental protection authority or other similar agencies for a list of approved experts to help mitigate the radon levels in the house. There are various methods which make it possible to lower the amount of radon to acceptable levels. Success depends on the likely sources of the radon gas, and on the technique used to lower the radon level.

PESTICIDES

It was found some time ago that farmers and other agricultural workers, who regularly use considerable amounts of insecticides, pesticides and weed killers, are more prone than is the general population to the development of certain malignant tumours, such as some lymphomas, and cancers of the prostate, skin, lung, and possibly leukaemias and soft tissue sarcomas.

There has been little research on the ill-effects of extensive insecticide, pesticide, weed killer and defoliant use in the household in relation to the risk of cancer. However, for those who want to play it safe, there are ways of limiting their use around the home by using natural methods of cultivating the home garden and lawn. If chemical agents are used, use the minimum amount required, follow the instructions strictly, wear protective garments and gloves, keep children and pets away from these agents, and wash your hands thoroughly after use. These precautions are important for both outdoor and indoor use. These chemicals should be stored in a safe place, preferably outside the house, and well away from children and pets.

HOUSEHOLD CLEANERS, SOLVENTS AND OTHER CHEMICALS

Cleaning fluids contain benzene, which in the occupational setting can contribute to the development of leukaemia. Another agent is methylene chloride, which is present in many paint strippers and paints, and in experimental animals can cause lung cancer, cancer of the breast and brain. As is the case with insecticides and weed killers, little scientific research has been conducted in the household with cleaners, solvents and chemicals. It is wise to take precautions, namely to avoid the use of solvents and other similar agents whenever possible, use as little as possible, ventilate the house after use, wash hands and clothes after use, and store these agents in a safe place, away from children and pets.

ELECTROMAGNETIC FIELDS (EMF)

Wherever there is electrical power, there is the possibility of both children and adults being exposed to low frequency electromagnetic fields (EMF). It is possible that prolonged exposure to this type of radiation is a factor in the development of some malignant tumours, particularly leukaemias, lymphomas and brain tumours.

In the early 1980s it was suggested that children exposed to EMF from residential proximity to high current power lines were more prone to brain tumours and leukaemias and possibly to lymphomas than would otherwise be expected. However, a recent large US study suggests that there may not be a risk present. It was also suggested that the prolonged use of electric blankets, a source of radio-frequency electromagnetic radiation, was associated more frequently than expected with leukaemias, and with cancers of the testicle. Subsequently, it was also found that electronic or electrical workers such as electricians, radio and TV repair technicians, telephone mechanics and computer mechanics, were more prone to leukaemias, lymphomas and brain tumours than would be expected. Research is currently underway for a possible link between brain cancer and the use of cellular phones. More recently, a possible link between these tumours in children who have residential proximity to cellular telephone towers has also been raised in Australia.

Although scientists are not in agreement regarding the role of EMF in the development of certain cancers, to be on the safe side it would be wise to stop children from playing near overhead power lines and cellular telephone towers. Whilst scientists are deliberating, it would also be wise not to be too close to the television set, not to make a habit of sleeping on electric blankets, and to avoid the excessive use of household appliances such as hairdryers, electric shavers, electric can openers, and whenever possible to keep as far away as possible from these appliances. The jury is still out on the induction of brain cancers by the use of cellular telephones. The main reason for keeping away from electric power lines and various appliances is that the strength of EMF dissipates very quickly when one moves away from the source.

HOW SAFE IS THE HOME ENVIRONMENT?

The chances are that one's home is safe. However, if there is concern about passive smoking, the presence of asbestos fibre or radon gas, or of electromagnetic fields in or around the house, or if pesticides, insecticides, weed killers, household cleaners, solvents and other chemicals have been used excessively and without due protection, now is the time to check these out and eliminate or minimise the risk by appropriate action.

> *Once everything has been done to protect the house, and it has been turned into a 'castle', enjoy it, the garden, family and friends to the full. This will give you great pleasure, and it may also further improve the chances of remaining in good health and free from cancer.*

PART III

PREVENTION AND EARLY DETECTION OF INDIVIDUAL CANCERS

14

Large bowel cancer
Cancer of the colon and rectum

Large bowel cancer (also called *colorectal cancer*, or *colon cancer* if it involves the first part of the large bowel, or *rectal cancer* if it involves the last part of the large bowel) is one of the commonest cancers in developed countries.

LARGE BOWEL STRUCTURE AND FUNCTION

The large bowel, the last part of the gastrointestinal tract or gut, is essentially a conducting tube. It is situated in the abdomen and pelvis, and its position in the body is shown in Figure 5.

The large bowel consists of four concentric layers, the innermost of which is called the *mucosa*. This is a lining layer of cells, and almost all tumours of the large bowel arise from this lining layer. The outer layers are composed of muscle and connective tissue.

The large bowel absorbs some water and minerals, but its main function is the storage and regular elimination of undigested food, mainly dietary fibre, bacteria and water. The large bowel is not an essential organ for human survival, as one can

Figure 5: The position of the large bowel in the body

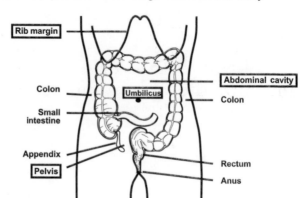

lead a reasonably normal life after the entire large bowel has been surgically removed.

ABOUT COLORECTAL CANCER

During 1999 it is expected that more than 750,000 individuals in the world will be diagnosed with colorectal cancer, and of these, about 150,000 will reside in the USA, over 30,000 in the United Kingdom, and about 10,000 in Australia. This cancer is common in both sexes, and almost half of those diagnosed with colorectal cancer are women.

The growth and spread of colorectal cancer

Colorectal cancer is one of the many cancers which develop in several steps from a normal lining cell of the mucosa, to cells which look abnormal when examined under the microscope, but which are not tumour cells (*hyperplasia* and *dysplasia*). From these abnormal cells the next stage in most instances is the development of a benign tumour called an *adenoma* (one type of bowel polyp), which is a precancerous condition, and from which an early locally invasive cancer develops. In some instances, the invasive cancer develops without the adenoma stage.

The earliest cancer stage, Stage A, is when the cancer is localised to the lining layer of the bowel. The next stage, Stage B, refers to a cancer which has spread through all layers of the large bowel. Stage C represents spread or metastasis to lymph glands adjacent to the bowel, whilst the most advanced is Stage D, in which the cancer has spread to distant organs, most commonly the liver.

What is the outlook for a person with colorectal cancer?

Only four of every ten individuals who develop colorectal cancer will survive to live a normal lifespan, while the other six will die prematurely from the effects of the cancer. However, if colorectal cancer is identified at an early stage, and before it has spread from the area of the mucosal lining (Stage A), then in nine out of ten instances the person will survive and live out their life normally.

EARLY SYMPTOMS AND ABNORMAL SIGNS

In many instances, there are no early warning symptoms or signs of colorectal cancer, nor of the main precancerous condition, colorectal adenomatous polyps. This is one of the reasons why it is important to undergo regular checkups along the lines recommended in this chapter, particularly in those who are 50 years of age or older. In some, bleeding with bowel motions, changes in the usual bowel habit, abdominal pain, abdominal tightness or distension may appear as warning signs, and these require early medical attention.

COLORECTAL CANCER—A MODEL FOR CANCER PREVENTION

Due to a great surge of enthusiasm among researchers all over the world during the past 20 years concerning the causes of colorectal cancer, and due to the major advances in the primary prevention and screening of this cancer, we now know that colorectal cancer could be largely eliminated within the next generation. The important causes are inherited factors, a certain type of diet, excessive alcohol consumption, smoking and physical inactivity. It is very interesting that all these causes apply not only to colorectal cancer, but also to the precancerous condition of colorectal adenomas, or polyps, from which two-thirds of all colorectal cancers develop. Three avenues of research, namely a better understanding of the causes, an improved knowledge of the cell changes from normal to a colorectal cancer cell, and the advent of effective screening tests have been particularly important in advancing our knowledge of how colorectal cancer may be prevented, or at least detected at an early and curable stage.

CAUSES OF COLORECTAL CANCER

In most instances of large bowel cancer the causes are known, or at least strongly suspected. This means that reversing those causes, that is, employing primary prevention, is likely to result in a marked decrease in the number of individuals who develop bowel cancer. Moreover, by knowing the high risk groups, it is also possible to perform screening tests for the early detection of cancer in these groups. The following is known about the causes of colorectal cancer.

Inherited causes

This is an important cause in about 15% (1 in 6) of those who develop bowel cancer. The uncommon family syndromes of familial adenomatous polyposis (FAP) and hereditary non-polyposis colorectal cancer (HNPCC) which together account for about 5% of all new instances of colorectal cancer, are described in detail in Chapter 4. The methods of early detection of cancer in family members of FAP and HNPCC, including the place of the recently available genetic blood tests, are described later in this chapter.

About 10% of those who develop colorectal cancer and who do not belong to FAP and HNPCC families are thought to have a hereditary cause, as gleaned from a history of colorectal tumours in near relatives. The genes that might be responsible for these cancers are at present unknown, with the possible exception of the subgroup of Ashkenazi Jews, who have been known to be at an increased risk for colorectal cancer for some time. Recently at the Johns Hopkins University Medical School Oncology Center, a gene mutation named I1307K has been identified, which is found among Ashkenazi Jews and which may be the inherited link for this subgroup of people at risk—a most exciting finding.

Dietary causes

Dr Ernst Wynder in New York and Dr Denis Burkitt (of 'Burkitt Lymphoma' fame) in England, pioneers of the 'dietary hypothesis of cancer' were the first to suggest in the 1960s that too much animal fat (Dr Wynder) and too little dietary fibre (Dr Burkitt) may be nutritional causes of colorectal cancer. Since then there has been overwhelming scientific evidence derived from many parts of the world which consistently suggests that diet is the important cause in about half of those who develop colorectal cancer. The type of diet which predisposes to this cancer is a high-calorie diet, which includes a high fat intake and a high sugar intake, a high consumption of meat, particularly red meat, a high consumption of animal fat, and a low consumption of vegetables, fruit and cereals, which means that there is also a low consumption of total dietary fibre. A low consumption of fish, and a low intake of calcium-containing foods, and a high intake of salt may be additional dietary causes of this common cancer. Being overweight or obese, a characteristic of those who have eaten a high-calorie diet for many years, and who are often also inactive, is a further risk for large bowel cancer. These are also the diet risks for the precancerous colorectal adenomas.

Alcohol consumption

For men, drinking three or more alcoholic drinks per day, or two or more drinks per day for women, for 20 or more years, and particularly if the main drink is beer, is important in about 10% of those who develop colorectal cancer. The risk appears to be greater for rectal cancer than for colon cancer. The alcohol risk is also present for the precancerous colorectal adenomas.

Smoking

Smoking is known to be an important cause of several cancers, such as cancer of the lung, throat, gullet, bladder, pancreas and others. It has only been in the last decade that scientists have discovered that smoking is also an important cause of colorectal adenoma, the benign tumour which is the main precancerous condition for colorectal cancer. It has been estimated that about 10% of colorectal cancers can be attributed to smoking.

Physical inactivity

A sedentary lifestyle in which little or no physical activity takes place appears to predispose an individual to the development of colon cancer.

CHANGES FROM THE NORMAL CELL TO A COLORECTAL CANCER ARE KNOWN

About two-thirds of all colorectal cancers start in a benign tumour, an *adenoma* or *adenomatous polyp*, and one-third become a cancer from a normal cell without going through the stage of an adenomatous polyp. However, only about 1 in 20 adenomas become a cancer, so that 95% of adenomatous polyps remain harmless. The term *'polyp'* merely refers to a lump on a stalk protruding from the lining of organs, such as the colon, rectum or cervix. A colorectal polyp can also be the result of inflammation, and then it is called a *hyperplastic* or *inflammatory polyp*. The distinction between adenomatous polyps and hyperplastic or inflammatory polyps is important because inflammatory or hyperplastic polyps are not precancerous conditions, and those who have had such a polyp removed in the past usually do not require follow-up, in contrast to those who have had adenomatous polyps removed, and who do require further follow-up.

The length of time it takes a normal cell to change to an adenomatous polyp and then to a colorectal cancer is quite long, and can be up to 30 years, although the usual time in most individuals is about ten years. This knowledge is important, because if we can systematically remove all adenomatous polyps, we would be able to prevent about two-thirds of all colorectal cancers. Moreover, repeated checkups of those who have had an adenomatous polyp removed (and because those with a previous adenoma are known to be at an increased risk of developing further adenomatous polyps), need not usually be more often than every three years, and in some cases, not more often than every five years, provided there is certainty that the initial adenomas were completely removed.

EFFECTIVE EARLY DETECTION USING SCREENING TESTS IS AVAILABLE

There are several effective tests available which can detect colorectal tumours, either adenomas or early cancers. These tests are *digital rectal examination, occult blood testing of the stool, flexible sigmoidoscopy, colonoscopy* and *barium enema examination*. These tests and when they are to be used, are described below. At present the main problem with systematic screening of the whole population is the high cost to the individual, and to the entire community.

COULD YOU DEVELOP COLORECTAL CANCER?

A personal risk list

The list in Table 14.1 provides an indication of whether an increased risk for colorectal cancer is present or not. However, I emphasise that most people who have one or more of these risk factors will *not* develop colorectal cancer during their lifetime. This check list merely means that if the 'yes' column is ticked one or more times, the best advice is to take action

Table 14.1: Risk factors for colorectal cancer

Due to inherited cancer risk	Yes	No
One or more near relatives with colorectal cancer One or more near relatives with colorectal adenomas (adenomatous polyps) Family members known to have hereditary syndromes of familial adenomatous polyposis (FAP), or hereditary non-polyposis colorectal cancer (HNPCC), sometimes also called Lynch syndromes I and II		
Due to personal health risks		
Colorectal cancer previously removed Colorectal polyps or adenomas previously removed History of ulcerative colitis or Crohn's disease History of previous breast cancer, uterine cancer, or ovarian cancer Past radiation treatment to the pelvis		
Due to personal lifestyle risks		
Undesirable diet (high in calories, fat, meat, salt; low in vegetables, fruit, cereals, fibre, fish) Overweight and obese (more than 20% over the desirable weight). Check desirable weight from Table 5.3. Alcohol (men consuming 3 or more drinks, women 2 or more drinks per day, especially beer, for several years) Smoking Inactive lifestyle		

which is likely to lower the chances of developing cancer of the colon or rectum.

This inventory of risk factors in an individual has been divided into two groups. The first group is *higher than average risk*, which means that they do have one or more specific risks which are known to be associated with an increased chance of developing colorectal cancer. In general, the risk rises the more often the 'yes' column has been ticked. The second group is called *average risk*, which means that this person does not have any known or specific risk factors. It is not called *low risk* because our Western lifestyle is such that we are at a higher risk than some traditional cultures in Asia, Japan and Africa, who are truly at low risk for cancer of the large bowel.

An 'average risk' individual for colorectal cancer is a person who did not tick any of the 'yes' boxes in Table 14.1, and is 50 years of age or older. If one or more 'yes' boxes were ticked, a person is at higher than average risk.

Primary prevention of colorectal cancer

Dietary changes, moderation of alcohol consumption, smoking cessation, a regular physical activity programme, and possibly the regular use of aspirin, are the main weapons in the primary prevention of colorectal cancer.

Is there conclusive scientific evidence that dietary change, alcohol moderation, smoking cessation and regular physical activity will substantially decrease the chances of developing colorectal cancer for an individual? The evidence, though not totally conclusive, is regarded as sufficiently strong for several national anticancer organisations, including the World Health Organization Collaborating Center for the Prevention of Colorectal Cancer, to make recommendations now. This advice, if put into practice, has no side-effects, and it is not harmful in any way to humans. Moreover, the recommendations are almost identical to the advice given for the prevention of chronic heart disease and artery disease, adult onset diabetes, and also for the promotion of a healthy lifestyle in general. So there is nothing to lose and there is likely to be a lot to be gained by following these recommendations.

Dietary change

No other cancer better illustrates the benefits of the type of diet recommended in a cancer prevention programme in Chapter 5, than does colorectal cancer. This is a cancer in which inappropriate diet, when consumed over many years, appears to be the most important single risk factor. The type of diet which is likely to lower the risk of colorectal cancer and also of the precancerous colorectal adenoma, will be one in which the total daily calories do not exceed 2500 for men, and 2000 calories for women, in which a lot of vegetables, plenty of bread, pasta, rice, cereals and fruit are eaten, and in which the fat consumption is reduced to 20% of the daily calories. Fish is eaten regularly, as is skinless chicken. Low-fat or non-fat dairy products are eaten to obtain protein and a high calcium intake. Lean meat is eaten infrequently, and heavily fried and grilled meat is avoided. Guidelines and tips on how to achieve this diet successfully appear in Chapter 5. It is especially important to eat plenty and a wide variety of vegetables, particularly cruciferous vegetables (cabbage, cauliflower, broccoli, brussel sprouts, swede, turnip, kohlrabi and kale), and to include yellow and green vegetables, since a high and varied vegetable intake appears to be the most important single component in the nutritional prevention of colorectal cancer. There is also good recent evidence from Australian research that over and above this diet, for those who have had adenomatous polyps removed in the past, the addition of a quarter of a cup of unprocessed wheat bran each day considerably reduces the chances of developing further adenomas.

Alcohol consumption

Recent research strongly suggests that limiting alcohol consumption to three alcoholic drinks per day for a man, and to two drinks per day for a woman, is likely to be useful in lowering the risk for colorectal cancer, and of the precancerous colorectal adenoma. For reasons that are not clear, beer is an at-risk beverage for colorectal tumours, whilst wine poses the least important alcohol risk. However, it would still be wise not to drink more than three glasses of wine per day for men and not more than two glasses per day for women.

Smoking

Smoking seems particularly important in the development of colorectal adenomas, the benign tumours from which two-thirds of all colorectal cancers develop. Quitting smoking can be difficult, and practical methods of smoking cessation are discussed in Chapter 6.

Physical activity

If your medical practitioner approves, performing 30 minutes or more of moderate physical activity five or more days per week is recommended, as among its other known health benefits, regular exercise may also decrease the risk of colon cancer and of the precancerous colon adenoma. 'Moderate' physical activity means doing something that raises the pulse and makes one sweat a little, such as brisk walking, gentle jogging, cycling, swimming or gymnasium work. This programme may also lower the risk for many other diseases, such as heart disease, and is also likely to improve vitality and one's sense of well-being.

Aspirin as a preventive

In 1988 my research group at the University of Melbourne had an exciting 'world-first' to report. Our studies showed that the regular use of aspirin was powerful as a preventive in both men and women, for both colon and rectal cancer. This finding has now been confirmed several times by studies in the USA, UK and elsewhere. In other recent studies, the same protection has also been found for the precancerous adenomatous polyp. The problems at present with regular aspirin use as a colorectal tumour preventive are that the optimum dose of aspirin to be used is not certain, and also that prolonged aspirin use may have undesirable side-effects in some individuals, particularly the possibility of bleeding from the bowel. Modified forms of aspirin are now being developed which may eliminate these undesirable side-effects of prolonged aspirin use. Some physicians in the USA have already suggested the use of one regular aspirin tablet (300 mg) every alternate day in those who are at a reasonably high risk for developing colorectal cancer, such as individuals who have a family history of bowel cancer. The results of controlled studies of long-term aspirin use, which are presently being conducted in the United Kingdom and the USA, and which will assess all the possible benefits (including protection from colorectal cancer), and all the potential harmful effects of regular aspirin use, are likely to resolve these problems. However, the currently available evidence suggests that aspirin, either in its present form or in some modified form, is likely to have an important future role in the primary prevention of colorectal cancer. *For the present, the best advice is to first discuss the wisdom of long-term aspirin use with a medical practitioner before embarking on this course of action.*

Hormone replacement therapy as a preventive

The prolonged use of hormone replacement therapy in post-menopausal women appears to confer significant protection against colorectal cancer. This is an unexpected benefit of hormone replacement therapy, over and above its other uses, such as the treatment of menopausal symptoms, or the prevention of osteoporosis.

EARLY DETECTION USING SCREENING TESTS

There are several effective screening tests available for the early detection, then removal, of both colorectal cancer, and its main precancerous condition, colorectal adenomatous polyps. Giving physician-directed advice to individuals in Western countries on the early detection of colorectal cancer using screening tests will be the main focus of this section. There is controversy regarding mass or population screening, mainly because of the high cost to the community. It is likely that for mass screening of colorectal cancer, each country will need to decide what will be the most appropriate method of screening, and this will be mainly governed by its economic and health priorities.

Screening tests for colorectal cancer

Digital rectal examination

This simple examination involves the gloved and lubricated finger of the medical practitioner inserted into the lower half of the rectum, a part of the large bowel in which many cancers arise. In practice the finger can reach up to 8–10 cm (3–4 inches), and can detect about 10% of all colorectal cancers. This test is usually uncomfortable, but not painful. It is completely safe, requires no preparation beforehand, and can reliably identify a cancer or a polyp. The presence of a cancer or polyp is then confirmed by doing a *biopsy,* which involves taking a piece or the whole of the tumour for examination under the microscope by a pathologist.

Occult blood in the stool

Many adenomatous polyps and many though not all bowel cancers bleed from time to time. This type of bleeding usually produces only traces of blood which cannot be seen by the naked eye when inspecting the stool. Because this blood is often invisible, the test which is used to detect it is called *faecal occult blood testing* (FOBT). This test usually involves taking stool samples for three consecutive days. Some of the stool is smeared onto a card, or placed into a container, and as per the instructions, it is returned to the doctor or the relevant laboratory.

Certain dietary precautions may be necessary and these will be indicated in the instructions.

The problem with faecal occult blood tests which are currently available is the relatively high number of *false negative tests* (colorectal tumour present, but the FOBT result is negative), as well as some *false positive tests* (colorectal tumour not present, but the FOBT is positive). While false negative tests miss tumours, false positive tests not only cause anxiety, but also lead to unnecessary invasive tests, in particular colonoscopy, as well as adding considerably to the total cost of screening. Although the number of reported false positive and false negative FOBT results varies in different studies, a reasonable prediction is that FOBT will miss tumours in about 1 of 4 (25%) individuals, and that about 1 of 20 (5%) with a positive FOBT will have a colonoscopy unnecessarily, because a tumour is not actually present. Because of these false positive and false negative results, FOBT is not a diagnostic test in its currently available forms. At present FOBT is only used for the screening of average risk, symptomless individuals, with the understanding that tumours in some will be missed and that some others will have an unnecessary colonoscopy. The reliability of FOBT in the detection of large bowel tumours is constantly being improved with the development of newer tests, so that ultimately we should have a stool blood test which is very reliable in identifying a bowel tumour.

The faecal occult blood test is not appropriate if bowel symptoms are already present, because of the relatively high rate of false negative tests. In these circumstances more accurate tests are needed, such as colonoscopy. While it has limitations because of the false negative tests in which tumours are missed, and some false positive tests requiring colonoscopy unnecessarily, it is important to realise that screening using the faecal occult blood test in large controlled studies conducted in the USA, UK and Scandinavia, has been able to reduce the number of premature deaths due to colorectal cancer by about 15%. The widespread use of FOBT is now being considered for mass screening by several governments in the Western world.

Flexible sigmoidoscopy

Screening experts increasingly recommend that faecal occult blood tests should be followed by flexible sigmoidoscopy. This is a flexible fiberoptic instrument that can go round the corners of the large bowel, and if there are no technical difficulties, it provides an excellent view of the lining of the bowel, up to 60 cm (24 inches) from the anus, as shown in Figure 6.

Provided the bowel is not full of stool, and provided there are no technical difficulties, flexible sigmoidoscopy can identify all colorectal cancers and adenomatous polyps up to 60 cm from the anus. Two-thirds of all cancers are located in this part of the large bowel. It is a safe office or outpatient procedure, requiring

Figure 6: Flexible fiberoptic sigmoidoscope fully inserted into the rectum and last part of the colon, which reaches to 60 cm (24 inches) from the anus

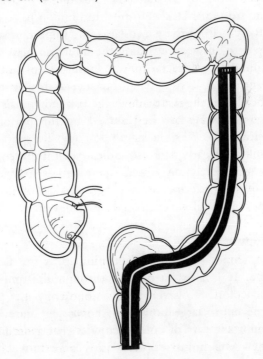

a fairly simple preliminary bowel preparation to empty the lower part of the large bowel. Complications from this procedure are most uncommon, and a perforation of the bowel has been reported in less than 1 of 5000 consecutive tests. Provided the bowel is empty, it is a very accurate method of detecting colorectal cancers and colorectal adenomas up to the part of the large bowel to which the flexible sigmoidoscope can be passed.

Controversial and currently unanswered questions are firstly whether to recommend screening flexible sigmoidoscopy after FOBT, irrespective of the FOBT result, and secondly whether to perform flexible sigmoidoscopy as the first screening test, thus omitting faecal occult blood testing entirely. In order to answer the first question of FOBT plus flexible sigmoidoscopy, a large controlled study was commenced by the National Cancer Institute in Bethesda USA in 1993, with final results to be reported in the year 2008. To answer the second question, whether to use flexible sigmoidoscopy as the only screening test, a large study coordinated from St Mark's Hospital in London has commenced recently. Results from these two large and important studies will provide us with answers regarding the direction mass or population screening for colorectal tumours will take us in the future. In the meantime, analysis of data from several smaller studies than those of the above, suggest that average risk individuals who wish to undergo screening are best served by the performance of FOBT followed by flexible sigmoidoscopy, irrespective of the FOBT result. The early data also indicate that if this combination is used as mass screening among symptomless individuals over the age of 50 in Western countries, a 30% reduction in premature death from colorectal cancer could be achieved.

Colonoscopy

The colonoscope is an instrument similar to the flexible sigmoidoscope. It is also introduced through the anus into the rectum and colon. However, with colonoscopy it is possible to examine the entire large bowel, as shown in Figure 7.

An important part of colonoscopy is that apart from being able to view the lining of the entire large bowel, it is also

Figure 7: The colonoscope fully inserted is able to view the lining of the entire colon and rectum

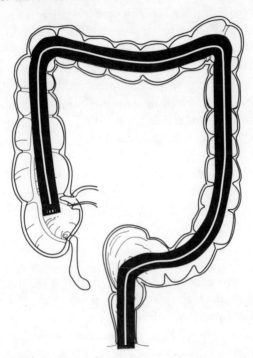

possible to take a piece of any abnormal tissue for biopsy and examination under the microscope. Thus it is possible to biopsy all polyps, tumours or any other suspicious lumps or swellings found on the lining of the large bowel. Before a colonoscopy is performed, the bowel needs to be prepared. There are certain dietary restrictions to follow as well as some special instructions, to make sure that the entire large bowel is empty at the time of the colonoscopy. This is all explained in the instructions given prior to the investigation. A short-acting sedative is usually given intravenously just prior to colonoscopy, so that those who have a colonoscopy have little recollection of the procedure.

A controversial question is why doesn't everyone who needs their large bowel screened have a colonoscopy as their first and only test? Although this view has been advanced by some physicians, so far it has not found general acceptance, partly because of the considerable cost and resources required if the entire population were to be screened and screened repeatedly by colonoscopy after the age of 50 years, and partly because there are some risks involved, namely the very occasional bowel perforation requiring surgical repair of the bowel, and the occasional excessive bleeding requiring blood transfusion. This procedure is also moderately demanding on the person under-going it, partly because of the bowel preparation necessary to get an empty bowel so that a good view is obtained, and partly because of the intravenous sedation which is necessary. Finally, it needs to be kept in mind that as a screening measure, colonoscopy would be done for those who are apparently well and without symptoms, and also that in most instances a bowel polyp or a bowel cancer would not in fact be found. In order to test the value of colonoscopy as the first and only screening investigation, physicians at the Memorial Sloan-Kettering Cancer Center in New York are planning to perform at a future time, a large controlled study of colonoscopy as the only screening test.

Colonoscopy, repeated at set intervals if used for the screen-ing of the entire population over 50 years of age would undoubtedly have the dramatic effect of largely eliminating colorectal cancer, because the entire large bowel could be carefully examined, and almost all polyps, adenomas and cancers found and removed. Because of the enormous cost as well as some slight risk which is associated with a colonoscopy, this is not practised at present. Colonoscopy, of course, is often used as the first investigation in the diagnosis of bowel symptoms, such as bleeding or a change in the bowel habit. However, colonoscopy, when performed for secondary prevention for the purposes of screening individuals who have no symptoms, is at present restricted to those who have a positive stool blood test, and also to certain very high risk groups, such as those with a very strong inherited predisposition to large bowel cancer, or those with longstanding ulcerative colitis.

Barium enema

This is a test done in a radiology department and it is performed by filling the large bowel with a liquid called *barium sulphate*, after the bowel has been previously cleaned out. Air is also injected later. This is called an *air contrast barium enema* and is more accurate than the ordinary barium enema. Barium enema examinations are very safe and much less expensive than colonoscopy. However, barium enemas are less accurate in finding small adenomatous polyps and small and early large bowel cancers than is colonoscopy. Also, biopsy of any abnormal polyp or suspicious lump or swelling cannot be done during a barium enema examination, and for this a colonoscopy needs to be performed. For these reasons, barium enema tests have been largely though not entirely superseded by colonoscopy.

RECOMMENDATIONS FOR SCREENING TESTS

These recommendations are guidelines only and it is best for every individual to discuss with their medical practitioner what is appropriate for them. The recommendations are divided into two main groups, namely those who have no known risk factors, the 'average risk' person, and those who have known risk factors, the 'higher than average risk' person.

Screening for average risk individuals

This group forms the majority of those screened for colorectal cancer. The term 'average risk' implies that these individuals are 50 years of age or older, and that they have no bowel symptoms and no known risk factors (as per Table 14.1, earlier in this chapter). In this category, the recommendations are to have:

- Annual digital rectal examination.
- Annual occult blood testing of the stool.
- Flexible sigmoidoscopy, first at age 50 and 5-yearly thereafter, whatever the occult blood test shows.

Screening for higher than average risk individuals

The description 'higher than average risk' describes those individuals who do not have symptoms of bowel cancer or of bowel polyps, may be at any age, and have one or more known risk factors, as indicated earlier in Table 14.1 in this chapter.

History of colorectal cancer or colorectal adenomas in one or more near relatives

Near relatives, sometimes called first-degree relatives, are parents, children, brothers and sisters. Uncles, aunts and grandparents, are not regarded as first-degree relatives.

If only one near family member has a history of colorectal cancer, then it is suggested that screening start at age 40, with stool blood testing annually and flexible sigmoidoscopy 3-yearly.

If two near relatives have colorectal cancer, or if a family member under age 45 years has a colorectal tumour, then stool blood testing annually and colonoscopy every three years, commencing at age 40 is recommended.

If three or more relatives have had bowel tumours, then hereditary non-polyposis cancer (HNPCC) is suspected, and the recommendations for screening in such situations are discussed shortly.

Familial adenomatous polyposis (FAP) known or suspected

The gene causing FAP is a mutation on chromosome 5, named the *adenomatous polyposis coli gene* or *APC gene* (Chapter 4). Genetic testing using special tests became available in the early 1990s, and this was a major advance in the screening of family members. These tests were called *linkage studies* and *mutational assays*. Using these methods no false positive tests have so far been identified. However, it has become clear that these methods will miss 1 in 4 (25%) of those who possess the abnormal APC gene, and because of these false negative tests, new methods of testing those who are at risk for FAP have been evolved. The most promising of these new tests is called *monoallelic mutation analysis* (MAMA). In conjunction with other tests, MAMA is able to detect at least 19 of 20 (95%) of those who have FAP.

The best advice at present is that those at risk for FAP attend a special centre for genetic counselling and have genetic testing using blood tests. Before these tests became available it was not possible to identify those members of FAP families who would develop polyps, given that only half the children of a parent with FAP will develop the condition. If the genetic test is positive, then screening needs to start at the very early age of ten or fifteen years and be performed regularly after that. Initially screening involves fiberoptic sigmoidoscopy. In most large cities special centres undertake genetic counselling and screening tests for family members with FAP.

Hereditary non-polyposis colorectal cancer known or suspected in a family (HNPCC, sometimes also called Lynch syndromes I and II)

If HNPCC is suspected, it is best to attend a special centre for further advice and management. HNPCC is suspected if three or more near relatives give a history of colorectal cancer, if these cancers occur at a relatively young age, such as 40 or 45 rather than the usual age of 65, and when these cancers have been present in several generations.

The genes causing HNPCC are mutations of the *DNA mismatch repair genes,* MSH2, MLH1, PMS1 and PMS2 (Chapter 4). Genetic testing for HNPCC using special blood tests has become possible since the 1990s in highly specialised centres in some countries, and clearly this will become the most important method of screening in the future. The problems with genetic testing at present are firstly that while in FAP families there is only one gene responsible, in HNPCC there are four different genes which may be affected, and each family appears to have its own pattern of abnormal mutations. This means that these blood tests need to be devised individually for every HNPCC family. The second problem is that as in FAP families, false positive tests have not been so far identified, so when using the early methods of mutational analysis 1 in 2 (50%) of those with

HNPCC will be missed. To overcome this high number of false negative tests, additional tests have been recently developed, including MAMA, as described for FAP, which together with other tests can now identify most individuals who have HNPCC. The testing of HNPCC families is therefore extremely time consuming and expensive.

If genetic testing is not available for members of HNPCC families, and for those who had positive genetic tests, colonoscopy commencing at the age of 25 and then performed every two years, and annual colonoscopy after the age of 35 is recommended. Additionally, members of HNPCC families also need to be carefully checked for other cancers, in particular for cancers of the uterus and ovary, and also cancers of the urinary system, the stomach and the pancreas.

Colorectal cancer or colorectal adenoma successfully removed previously

These individuals are at a higher risk of developing further bowel tumours, and for this reason colonoscopy performed every three years is recommended at present. Research increasingly suggests that if only a small adenoma was found initially, then colonoscopy every five years, or even flexible sigmoidoscopy every five years may be sufficient. However, until this issue is clarified, it is safest at present to recommend 3-yearly colonoscopy for all who have had either an adenomatous polyp or a colorectal cancer removed in the past.

Personal history of ulcerative colitis or of Crohn's disease

In a number of those who have either chronic ulcerative colitis or Crohn's disease, a part or the whole of the large bowel has been removed surgically. For those in whom the entire colon was removed, leaving only the rectum, screening would need to involve the use of flexible sigmoidoscopy only. Those who have had the entire colon and rectum removed, clearly do not need screening procedures, because there is no large bowel left to screen. For those who have not lost any part of their large bowel and who have had symptoms for eight years or longer, annual colonoscopy is recommended.

Previous breast, uterine and ovarian cancer

These women are at a higher than expected risk for developing colorectal cancer. Moreover, if they also had radiation in the pelvis for the treatment of uterine or ovarian cancer, their risk rises even higher. Annual stool blood testing and 3-yearly fiberoptic sigmoidoscopy is recommended. If the previous cancers were detected at a relatively young age, that is before 45, screening is best commenced at the age of 45 rather than age 50, as is currently recommended for the 'average risk' woman. Women who have also received pelvic radiation are recommended to commence screening at 45 years of age or five years after radiation, whichever comes first.

Previous pelvic radiation

Radiation to the pelvic area, given as treatment for any reason, increases the cancer risk for the lower large bowel, and this risk appears about five years after radiation has been given. Annual stool blood testing and 3-yearly fiberoptic sigmoidoscopy commencing five years after radiation is recommended.

Undesirable diet habits, excessive alcohol consumption, and smoking

As about two-thirds of all colorectal tumours appear to be linked to undesirable dietary habits, excessive alcohol consumption and smoking, those who have these risks are quite susceptible to developing bowel tumours. Although scientists so far have not made precise recommendations for the screening of these individuals, to be on the safe side this writer would recommend annual stool blood testing and flexible sigmoidoscopy commencing at age 45 rather than age 50, and flexible sigmoidoscopy repeated every three years.

THE FUTURE FOR COLORECTAL CANCER PREVENTION AND SCREENING

Research strongly suggests that if recommendations for screening, similar to those described above, are put into place in a developed country, such as the USA, UK, France, Italy, Germany, Australia or New Zealand, then the number of individuals who develop colorectal cancer can be greatly reduced, and the death rate from this cancer can be halved. If added to these screening recommendations a large part of the population adopts healthy dietary habits, stops smoking, moderates their alcohol consumption, engages in regular physical activity, and possibly some at high risk use aspirin regularly also, then based on current scientific data, it has been predicted by many experts, including the author, that this cancer could be largely eliminated within the next generation.

15

Breast cancer

She unlaced her bosum to disclose
Each breast a rose

Robert Graves (1895–1985)

A woman's breasts are, for her, much cherished symbols of her femininity, sexuality and motherhood. It is sad when a woman needs to lose her breast, or even part of it, because she has developed breast cancer.

A week does not go by without news about recent developments in breast cancer detection and treatment. Prominent women, Mrs Betty Ford, wife of past US President Gerald Ford, and movie stars Shirley Temple, Ingrid Bergman and Olivia Newton-John have courageously acknowledged their cancer in public, and have inspired many other women to be positive in relation to the fight against cancer. Although much progress has been made, we are not nearly as well advanced in the prevention of breast cancer as we are, for instance, in the prevention of colorectal cancer or skin cancer. We should urge our policy makers to increase funding for research on the prevention and early detection of breast cancer.

ANATOMY OF THE FEMALE BREAST

The female breast is a gland which produces milk after child-birth, and it is also an important secondary sex characteristic of the adult woman. The breast consists of glandular tissue in several lobules or segments surrounded by connective tissue and fatty tissue. In fact, fat and connective tissue form a large part of the female breast. Each breast sits on chest wall muscles, and lies directly under the skin, as indicated in Figure 8.

Figure 8: The anatomy of the female breast

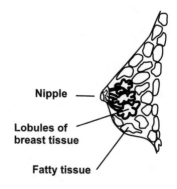

Nipple ———

Lobules of
breast tissue

Fatty tissue

ABOUT BREAST CANCER

Breast cancer is fortunately uncommon in women under 40 years of age, and less than 1 in 20 of all breast cancers develop before that age. However, the chances of developing breast cancer increase with age in those who are over 40 years old. Almost all breast cancers occur in women, and less than 1% occur in men. This chapter will be devoted entirely to breast cancer in women.

How common is breast cancer?

It has been estimated that in the United States a woman has about 1 chance in 10 of developing breast cancer during her

144

lifetime, and similar estimates have been made in other Western countries, such as Australia, New Zealand and the United Kingdom. Looking at this in a positive way, about 9 of 10 women in the USA, or about 90%, will *not* develop breast cancer. During 1999 about 800,000 women will develop breast cancer throughout the world, and of these, about 190,000 will occur in the USA, over 30,000 in the UK and about 8000 in Australia.

Growth and spread of breast cancer

Breast cancers, as do other cancers, enlarge by the multiplication of cancer cells. An *early breast cancer* has been defined as a tumour which is 2 cm (4/5th of an inch) in diameter, or smaller. Such a cancer is also referred to as a Stage I breast cancer. If cancer cells have travelled out of the breast, and into the lymph glands which drain the breast, such as the glands situated in the armpit or axilla, this is referred to as Stage II breast cancer. Further growth of the cancer so that it enlarges in size and becomes attached to the underlying muscle, and also when the cancer cells have enlarged considerably in the surrounding lymph glands, but there is no evidence of distant spread or metastasis, such as to the liver or lungs, is referred to as Stage III breast cancer. Stage IV breast cancer is the most advanced type, in which the cancer has spread far from the breast, such as when secondary or metastatic cancer is present in the liver, lung or brain.

What is the outlook for a woman with breast cancer?

A little more than half of all the women who develop breast cancer survive and live a normal lifespan. However, 6 out of 7 women (or about 85%) diagnosed with an early breast cancer, less than 2 cm (not quite 1 inch), and in whom the tumour has not spread outside the breast (Stage I), will survive and live a normal life after the cancer has been removed. Opposed to the excellent chances of a normal lifespan with a Stage I cancer, the chances of survival decrease with a Stage II breast cancer, and with Stage III and IV cancer, such as a large tumour which has been present for some years, and which has spread to the lymph glands or even further, the outlook is usually gloomy.

It is most important to identify a breast cancer early, so that it can be effectively treated, and with a high probability of curing the cancer.

EARLY SYMPTOMS AND ABNORMAL SIGNS

In early breast cancer, there may be no warning symptoms or signs, and this is one of the reasons why it is important to undergo regular examination as described later, particularly for a woman who is over 40 years of age. The most important early sign of breast cancer is feeling a lump or a thickening in the breast, or seeing a lump or thickening on a mammogram.

Discomfort or actual pain in the breast, or nipple discharge, are uncommon manifestations of early breast cancer. It is emphasised that often there are no warning symptoms of early breast cancer.

CAUSES OF BREAST CANCER

The causes of breast cancer are less well known than those of some other common tumours such as cancer of the lung, colon or rectum. Important contributory causes are inherited factors, diet, excessive alcohol consumption, hormonal changes, possibly physical inactivity, and uncommonly, excessive radiation to the chest.

Inherited breast cancer

An inherited tendency is important for about 1 in 4 women who develop breast cancer. The most important clue for an inherited predisposition to breast cancer is a history of breast cancer in one or more near relatives. This clue becomes more significant if breast cancer in the family has straddled several generations, and if breast cancer has developed at a relatively young age in a family member, such as at the age of 35 or 40 years. The problem with family history data is that many women who have a family history of breast cancer do not develop this cancer during their lifetime, while in others a reliable family history cannot be obtained. There is no family history of breast cancer in 75% of all women who develop that cancer.

The difficulties of obtaining an accurate family history of breast cancer have prompted molecular biologists to search for *genetic markers*, signposts of inherited breast cancer. Understandably, there was much jubilation when an abnormal gene named BRCA1 was identified a few years ago, and this was soon followed by the discovery of BRCA2, in which the preliminary data strongly suggested that these genes are genetic markers of inherited breast cancer. Moreover, the early data also suggested that the rare breast and ovarian cancer syndrome (BOCS) is strongly associated with the BRCA1 gene. The enthusiasm generated by these early results has been dampened by more recent studies from the USA and Australia which indicate that the lifetime risk of developing breast cancer in the presence of a BRCA gene is likely to be less than 85–90%, as suggested by the inital data. It has also been shown that some women who have a BRCA gene and develop breast cancer under the age of 40, do not have a family history of breast cancer.

The most important first clue to an inherited tendency for breast cancer at present, is a history of breast cancer in one or more near relatives, and especially so when such breast cancer developed at a relatively early age, such as 35 or 40 years of age, and when it occurs in several generations. A positive family history of breast cancer, together with an abnormal BRCA gene make it very likely that there is an inherited breast cancer risk. However, the precise level of that risk has not been clarified, and we await the results of further research, so that in the presence of either a positive or a negative genetic test, more accurate and more informative advice and recommendations can be made than is possible at present. Although gene testing is now available, in view of the uncertainty about its interpretation, women who have genetic testing should receive genetic counselling about its implications.

Dietary factors

Diet does appear to be a contributory cause of breast cancer also, although this has been much less clearly defined than has the role of diet in colorectal cancer. A diet high in calories, high in animal fat and meat, and low in vegetables, fruit, cereals and therefore low in fibre, appears to increase the risk of breast cancer. Among vegetables, cruciferous vegetables (cabbage, cauliflower, broccoli) appear to be important in prevention. A high consumption of foods containing beta-carotene and vitamin E, and foods containing calcium, appear to offer a degree of protection against breast cancer (Chapter 5). Moreover, postmenopausal women who are also overweight or obese are at an increased risk for breast cancer.

Excessive alcohol consumption

It is likely that more than two alcoholic drinks per day increases the risk of breast cancer.

Hormone changes

A hormonal basis for breast cancer has been suspected for some time. Women who have had their ovaries removed surgically have a *decreased* chance of developing breast cancer subsequently. Situations in which there is overexposure to oestrogens, such as in women who have an early onset of menstruation, or a later cessation of menstruation, or women who have not had children or had children at a late stage in their life, such as after 35 years of age, or women who have had an abortion, have a higher than average risk of developing breast cancer. In contrast, having children decreases breast cancer risk. Lactation and breast feeding, events which are associated with hormone changes, may also protect a woman against breast cancer, although this is not certain. Hormone replacement therapy (HRT) increases slightly the chances of developing breast cancer. Current research suggests that the overall benefits of HRT when used appropriately for menopausal symptoms or for the prevention of osteoporosis are probably greater than the risk of breast cancer. The use of the oral contraceptive pill is probably not a risk unless the person is predisposed to breast cancer for other reasons, such as having a close relative with breast cancer, and unless the woman is using the pill currently. Under such circumstances, the contraceptive pill increases the risk of breast cancer slightly.

Hormonal changes are an important cause of breast cancer, and the underlying common factor for this appears to be either an intermittent or a sustained elevation in oestrogen hormone levels.

Physical inactivity

A sedentary and inactive life is often associated with being overweight or obese, as well as with an undesirable diet. However, being physically inactive in itself adds to the risk of developing breast cancer.

Radiation

Female survivors of the Hiroshima and Nagasaki atomic explosions have developed breast cancer at a higher rate than would otherwise be expected. Also, women who have had a large number of chest x-rays or more complicated radiological tests to the chest over several years, have an increased risk for breast cancer. These data have led to a reduction in the radiation dose of mammography, so that mammography, as used at present, is most unlikely to be harmful.

FROM A NORMAL BREAST THROUGH PRECANCER TO CANCER

The abnormal changes in breast cells as they develop from a normal breast to a breast cancer are not as well known as these changes in some other cancers, such as in cancers of the colon or rectum. Breast cysts are common, although women with breast cysts are not at an increased risk. However, a practical problem for the medical practitioner is that breast cysts appear as lumps in the breast, as do breast cancers, and it may be difficult to identify an early breast cancer in women who also have cysts in the breast.

When the pathologist examines tissue from a breast biopsy under the microscope, there may be some cell changes which in themselves are not cancerous, but which are nevertheless a warning that this woman has an increased chance of developing breast cancer in the future, that is, these are precancerous conditions. These pathology changes relate to the duct tissue in the breast. The important precancerous cell changes are the presence of polyps in the ducts, called *papillomas,* or abnormal breast cells referred to as *hyperplasia* or *dysplasia*, now most commonly called *atypical hyperplasia*.

A PERSONAL RISK LIST FOR BREAST CANCER

The check list of risk for breast cancer is divided into two groups, namely women with 'higher than average risk', where one or more known risk factors are present, and 'average risk', which means that no known risk factors are present.

Higher than average risk women

The 'higher than average risk' woman has one or more known or suspected risk factors present. Having a risk factor does *not* mean that breast cancer will invariably develop, because in fact most women with a 'higher than average risk' do not develop breast cancer. It simply means that the woman needs to be aware that there is an increased risk of breast cancer, and that appropriate steps towards prevention and screening are recommended. The action which can be taken is described later in this chapter. A woman is at a 'higher than average risk' for breast cancer if one or more 'yes' boxes are ticked in Table 15.1.

Table 15.1: Risk factors for breast cancer

	Yes	No
Due to inherited cancer risk		
One or more near relatives have breast cancer Several relatives have breast and/or ovarian cancer Positive BRCA1 or BRCA 2 gene test		
Due to personal health risks		
Breast cancer previously removed Previous breast biopsy showed a *papilloma* or *breast hyperplasia* or *breast dysplasia* or *atypical hyperplasia* or *duct carcinoma in-situ* One or more of following hormone-related events: 1) Menstruation before age 12 and after age 50 2) No children or first child after age 35 3) Pregnancy aborted 4) Uses oral contraceptives now 5) Uses hormone replacement therapy Had radiation treatment to chest or numerous x-rays to chest		
Due to personal lifestyle risks		
Overweight or obese (more than 20% over desirable weight) *Check desirable weight from Table 5.3* Undesirable diet (high calories, high fat, low vegetables, fruit, cereals, starch, fibre and fish) Drinks more than 2 alcoholic drinks per day Physically inactive		

Average risk women

The 'average risk' woman does not have any known inherited, personal or lifestyle risks as indicated in Table 15.1. Such a person is called 'average risk' rather than 'low risk' because in Western communities, the rate of breast cancer is high compared to countries with traditional lifestyles, such as in some Asian and African cultures, or in Japan. An *average risk* woman for breast cancer is one who did not tick any of the 'yes' boxes in Table 15.1, and is 40 years of age or older.

PRIMARY PREVENTION OF BREAST CANCER

Dietary change, weight control, physical activity and moderation of alcohol consumption appear to be some of the factors which are likely to lower a woman's chances of developing breast cancer.

Dietary change

Decreasing total calories to no more than 2000 per day, reducing fat consumption to 20% of daily calories, eating a lot of vegetables, bread, pasta, rice, cereals and fruit, eating fish, skinless chicken, low-fat or non-fat dairy products and eating lean meat only occasionally, form the essence of a dietary cancer prevention programme for breast cancer. To achieve this successfully please review Chapter 5 which deals in detail with the dietary prevention of cancer.

Alcohol consumption

For regular alcohol consumers it is wise to limit daily alcohol intake to two standard drinks per day. It is also useful to have two or more alcohol-free days per week, and to drink low-alcohol content beverages on occasions. Chapter 7 describes alcohol-related cancers, and the methods of achieving moderation in alcohol consumption.

Physical activity

Provided a woman is medically and physically fit to perform this, 30 minutes or more of moderate physical activity five or more days per week so that the pulse goes up a little, doing activities such as brisk walking, gentle jogging, cycling, swimming or gymnasium work, may be useful not only in the prevention of breast cancer, but also in lowering the risk for many other illnesses, such as colorectal cancer and heart disease (Chapter 9). A recent Australian study has also shown that women who engage in regular physical activity as a hobby, tend to improve their sense of vitality and self-image.

Weight control

Being overweight or obese appears to be a risk for breast cancer in postmenopausal women. By following the type of diet recommended in this book (Chapter 5) and by performing regular physical activity (Chapter 9), normalisation of weight is likely to occur.

Chemoprevention with drugs and nutritional supplements

The use of a drug *tamoxifen* in the primary prevention of breast cancer, especially in women at a high risk for this cancer, is a practical possibility. However, controlled scientific studies need to be performed because of the possible risks and side-effects which may be present when this drug is used by women who are well and have no symptoms. Studies are proceeding in the USA, UK, Italy and Australia, in which women who are at a higher than average risk of developing breast cancer are receiving tamoxifen. The early results of the US study, released in 1998, are optimistic and have suggested that regular tamoxifen use can prevent the development of breast cancer in a significant number of women. The final results of these studies are eagerly awaited.

The possible beneficial effects of nutritional supplements

containing *vitamin E*, have been suggested in the primary prevention of breast cancer, but so far there have been no conclusive scientific studies showing a beneficial effect. For the present it is much better to eat plenty of vegetables, fruit and cereals which contain not only vitamin E, but also many other compounds which are known to have anticancer properties (Chapter 5). The role of nutritional and other supplements in cancer prevention is discussed in Chapter 5 also.

Hormone replacement therapy

The fear of developing breast cancer as a result of hormone replacement therapy (HRT) remains an unsolved problem at present. It is hoped that the results of ongoing major US and UK studies, in which the effects of HRT will be assessed in postmenopausal women, will provide some answers. The evidence up to now suggests that HRT slightly increases a woman's chances of developing breast cancer. Every woman needs to balance this slight increase in risk against the beneficial effects for which the HRT is being used, such as the relief of menopausal symptoms, or the prevention of cardiovascular disease and osteoporosis. The benefits and risks of HRT use are always best discussed with a medical practitioner, since the pros and cons of HRT use would vary according to the individual woman's health history.

Oral contraceptives

Numerous studies have found that oral contraceptive pill use is, overall, not a risk for the subsequent development of breast cancer. However, oral contraceptive pill use may pose a slight risk in the subgroup of women who started to use it in adolescence, and are current users, but probably only when there are some other risks present as well, such as heavy alcohol consumption. As with hormone replacement therapy, it is wise to discuss with one's medical practitioner, oral contraceptive use in relation to the risk of breast cancer.

Preventive bilateral simple mastectomy

This major operation, in which both breasts are removed as a preventive measure, would be recommended if the development of breast cancer is assessed to be inevitable. The problem is that at present the prediction of the precise chances of developing breast cancer in a particular person cannot be made with complete accuracy. Detailed explanation and discussion between the patient and her medical advisers, which should also include an expert second opinion, or a discussion of the case in front of an expert multidisciplinary panel are important, so that the woman can then make an informed choice.

Very occasionally, a woman has an extremely high chance of developing breast cancer because her health history includes several important risks, one of which almost always is a strong history of breast cancer in the family. A typical example would be a woman aged 48, whose mother and two sisters have had a breast cancer removed in the past. She has a positive BRCA1 gene test. She has also had three previous breast biopsies, the first of the left breast showing a duct papilloma, the second and third of the right breast, both showing high grade atypical hyperplasia. Moreover, she is also overweight, physically inactive, and has been a daily consumer of at least four alcoholic drinks for many years. Under such or similar unusual circumstances, the removal of both breasts may be considered. In this operation, all breast tissue must be removed, a procedure which can be technically difficult, particularly in the stage of the operation when the breast and duct tissue which lies directly under the nipple is being removed. In fact, it may be very difficult to be sure that all breast tissue has been removed. If some breast tissue is left behind, then the woman is still at some risk of developing breast cancer in the breast tissue which has not been removed. In this operation, the overlying skin and the nipple is usually left undisturbed, and only the breast tissue and surrounding fat is removed. It is usually recommended that breast implants be inserted.

Most women have coped well following these operations.

Preventive breast removal is uncommonly done, and to put it into perspective, in the writer's surgical practice, extending over a 30-year period in which consultation was sought by more than 3000 women with breast conditions, a preventive bilateral breast removal to avoid breast cancer was recommended on only three occasions.

EARLY DETECTION OF BREAST CANCER USING SCREENING TESTS

Breast self-examination, a breast check by a medical practitioner, and mammography, are the three important screening tests for breast cancer. Some women also have an ultrasound examination of the breast, usually as a diagnostic test. Ultrasound is not used for the screening of breast cancer at present. Breast biopsy will confirm or deny the presence of breast cancer. In the future, genetic testing using blood tests may also become available for those women who are at risk of developing inherited breast cancer. Genetic testing is an exciting future prospect in the early detection of breast cancer.

Screening tests for breast cancer

Breast self-examination (BSE)
Most breast lumps are discovered by women themselves, and this particularly applies to those women who have learned to examine their breasts regularly.

It cannot be emphasised too strongly that whilst most breast lumps and breast thickenings turn out not to be cancer, but rather an innocent swelling such as a breast cyst, once a breast lump is discovered, an expert medical examination and advice is essential.

Several studies have clearly shown that women who perform regular breast self-examinations are not only more likely to find breast lumps, some of which turn out to be a breast cancer, but also they are more likely to find small breast cancers at an early stage of their development, when they can be removed with a very high likelihood of permanent cure. Breast self-examination is simple, as may be seen from the diagrams and instructions which appear in Figure 9. In those women who are menstruating, the best time to examine the breasts is a few days after a period. In women who have stopped menstruating, choosing a regular day each month is a useful way to remember to examine the breasts.

The drawings and text in Figure 9 depict a commonly used method of breast self-examination. There are other similar methods of BSE, all of which are satisfactory, provided they have been demonstrated by an expert, and provided both breasts are examined carefully and completely.

Medical breast check

Regular and usually annual examination of the breasts by a medical practitioner is recommended for a woman over 40 years of age. Such an examination also needs to be done if something suspicious is found by a woman after breast self-examination, or in any other way. Medical practitioners have their own particular techniques of examining the breasts, although it is not unlike the breast self-examination method just described. The medical practitioner will also feel for the presence of any lymph glands situated in the armpits.

Mammography

This is an x-ray examination of the breasts which can often identify a small breast cancer even before it can be felt by self-examination or by a medical practitioner during a breast check. Systematic mammography of entire populations studied in Scandinavia and Holland has found that the chances of dying from breast cancer can be reduced by almost one-third,

Figure 9: Steps in breast self-examination

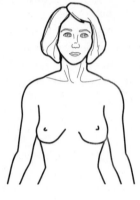

Standing in front of a mirror, inspect both breasts for any obvious swelling, dimpling or puckering of the breast skin or of the skin around the nipple.

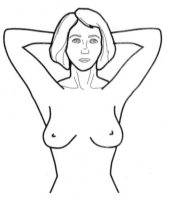

Raise the arms and this will change the tension and shape of the breast, and again look for any abnormal swelling, lumps, or puckering of the skin or nipples.

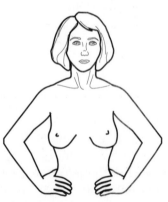

Still standing in front of a mirror, hands on hips, bend slightly forward towards the mirror and again look at the contour of the breasts.

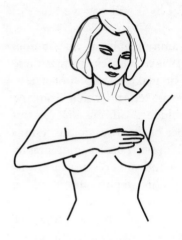

Now examine the wet breasts whilst under the shower or in a bath. Applying soap allows the fingers to glide more easily over the skin. This may make it easier to feel any abnormal lump or thickening. Use the right hand to feel the left breast while carefully going over the breast tissue in a rotatory manner. Repeat this with the right breast, using the left hand, again making sure that the whole breast is felt in this way.

Lying flat on the back, again feel the breasts with the fingers in a rotatory manner. This can be done first with the other arm by the side, and then raising the arm overhead, which flattens the breast. A pillow may be placed under the shoulder blade on the side of the breast being examined, but this is not essential. Repeat the procedure on the other breast, again making sure that the whole breast is felt in this way.

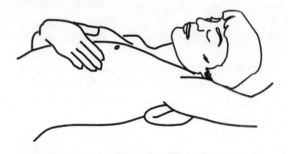

especially in women between the ages of 50 and 69 years. A government funded Australian national mammography screening programme, *BreastScreen Australia* has been in operation throughout the country since 1992. The preliminary outcome results are optimistic, and it is predicted that lives will be saved by this screening programme.

One of the shortcomings of mammography is that it does not detect a breast cancer in about 10% of women, so that these false negative results certainly do not make it a foolproof test. Also, mammography will disclose breast lesions which from the mammogram appearance cannot exclude a cancer, and for this reason a biopsy is required. A number of these suspicious lesions are shown not to be a cancer on biopsy. Thus mammography can also result in unnecessary anxiety and unnecessary intervention. Improvements in mammographic techniques, and in particular the future use of computer-aided mammography and computer analysed mammograms, may help the radiologist to improve the accuracy of interpretation, so that screening mammograms will find more early breast cancers than they do with methods used currently.

> *In spite of some false negative results of mammography, it should be remembered that if a breast cancer is detected by screening mammography, the chances of living a normal lifespan after its surgical removal are much better than waiting until it can be felt by a doctor.*

Mammograms are performed in a radiology department, and the best results are obtained using specially designed equipment. It has been found that mammogram films examined by two radiologists independently produce more accurate results. The breast is placed, and to some extent compressed between two plates, and two x-ray films are taken of each breast. The procedure can be uncomfortable and may cause transient breast pain, especially in women who have small breasts.

Breast biopsy
If a lump, swelling or thickening is felt in the breast, a piece of it can be removed and sent to a pathologist for microscopic

examination. This is the only way in which a breast cancer can be identified accurately. There are various ways of performing a biopsy, and the simplest is called *fine needle aspiration biopsy/cytology*. In this test, a local anaesthetic is given and the surgeon introduces a fine needle on a syringe into the breast and into the breast lump. If the lump is a cyst and contains fluid, all the fluid is sucked back by the syringe. If the lump is solid, then a piece of tissue is sucked back into the needle. If the aspiration reveals that the swelling is due to fluid only, and the lump disappears completely after the procedure, the woman can be reassured it is not a cancer, and nothing further needs to be done. If it is a solid lump, then the piece of tissue in the needle is squirted onto a slide and sent to a pathologist for a cytology examination. With solid lumps, a bigger piece of tissue may be required. In this case a core biopsy can be performed, still using a needle but of a larger bore than is used for aspiration biopsy. This is called a *needle-core biopsy*. Needle biopsies are performed under local anaesthesia in an office or clinic, and it is possible for the woman to leave immediately after the procedure.

False positive tests, that is, the result is returned as positive for breast cancer but in fact there is no breast cancer present, do not usually occur with a needle biopsy. *False negative tests,* that is, the result is returned as negative for breast cancer but in fact there is a cancer present in that breast, can occur with a needle biopsy, when the needle misses the cancer and removes an adjacent piece of non-cancerous tissue. Thus, a needle biopsy result which is positive for cancer is almost always accurate, but a needle biopsy result which is negative for cancer is not always accurate.

Sometimes the entire lump needs to be removed by a surgical procedure, and this is now usually performed as a day procedure using a general anaesthetic. A small cut is made over the swelling and usually the entire lump is removed. This is called a *surgical biopsy*. Sometimes a surgical biopsy is aided by using x-rays to find a small lump, and this method has been extremely useful for finding and removing small breast cancers which could not be felt and which were seen only on a mammogram. A surgical biopsy, especially when the whole lump is removed, almost always accurately determines whether the lump removed is or is not a breast cancer.

Genetic testing

As discussed earlier in this chapter, recent studies in the USA and Australia have indicated that blood tests which reveal the abnormal genes BRCA1 and BRCA2 are not linked with the subsequent development of breast cancer as often as had been suggested by the early studies, and also that some women who develop breast cancer under the age of 40 do not in fact have a family history of breast cancer. Those whose BRCA tests are positive will not necessarily develop breast cancer during their lifetime, while those whose BRCA tests are negative may still be predisposed to inherited breast cancer. Further research is ongoing to clarify the place of genetic testing for inherited breast cancer.

RECOMMENDATIONS FOR SCREENING

Australia is one of only a few countries in the world which funds a national mammography screening programme, *BreastScreen Australia*. This programme actively recruits women who are over 50 years of age for 2-yearly screening mammography. Women who are 40–49 and over 75 years of age are not actively recruited, but are welcome to attend free of charge, on their own initiative, for 2-yearly screening.

The recommendations which appear below should be taken as guidelines only. It is always important for each woman to discuss individually with her medical practitioner, the best means of screening for breast cancer. The recommendations for screening which follow refer only to women who seek breast cancer screening which is doctor-directed, and not for mass screening.

Recommendations are made for two distinct groups of women. The first are those who have no known risk factors, whom we have described earlier as *average risk* women, and the second are those women who have known risk factors, such as an inherited tendency for breast cancer, and are therefore at a *higher than average risk*. Please review Table 15.1 in this chapter, which summarises the several risk factors for breast cancer.

Average risk women, no breast symptoms

The majority of women screened for breast cancer belong to the 'average risk' group. This implies that these women have no breast symptoms and have no known risk factors, as indicated previously in Table 15.1. The specific recommendations for this group appear in Table 15.2.

Table 15.2: Screening average risk women for breast cancer

Women aged 20–39
- 3-monthly breast self-examination (BSE)
- 3-yearly medical breast check

Women aged 40 and over
- Monthly BSE
- Yearly medical breast check
- Baseline mammogram age 40, then 2 yearly

Screening of 'higher than average risk' women with no breast symptoms

Having one or more risk factors as summarised in Table 15.1 would put a woman into a higher than average risk category for breast cancer. Examples of increased risk include a near relative with breast cancer, a previously removed breast cancer, previous breast biopsy showing a precancerous condition, or being markedly overweight with an undesirable diet. In this group of women it is usually wise to commence screening mammography at age 40, or immediately if the woman is already over the age of 40. However, if there is a family history of breast cancer, start screening mammography ten years before the youngest family member was first diagnosed, or at age 40, whichever comes first. Also, if the woman has had a breast cancer or a precancerous breast condition previously removed, start screening mammography at the time of diagnosis. The specific recommendations for women who are at higher than average risk for breast cancer appear in Table 15.3.

Table 15.3: Screening higher than average risk women for breast cancer

Women aged 40 and over
- Monthly BSE
- Yearly medical breast check
- Yearly mammography

Please see text for age of commencement under certain special circumstances

---

THE FUTURE FOR BREAST CANCER SCREENING AND PREVENTION

Although much has been achieved, more research needs to be done to better understand the causes of breast cancer, so that more emphasis can be placed on primary prevention. Chemoprevention, particularly with the use of tamoxifen, may in the future be able to prevent breast cancer developing in some women. Screening tests and particularly mammography need to be refined further, so that they are more accurate. Hopefully also, more accurate genetic tests will become available for those who have an inherited tendency for breast cancer, so that effective screening tests can be instituted for these women. Education of women in primary prevention will no doubt lower the number of women who develop this cancer. Improvements in screening methods will detect more early breast cancers, and will improve the chances of living out a normal lifespan.

16

Lung cancer

Lung cancer has the dubious honour of being the leading cause of cancer deaths in many countries, including the USA, United Kingdom and Australia. It is also very high on the list of cancer deaths in other European countries, as well as in Japan, China, and some other Asian countries.

> *The main cause of lung cancer is smoking, so it should be easy to largely prevent this cancer by the avoidance of all tobacco use. However, this is not the reality, as many will not give up the smoking habit, even though it is known that regular smokers have a 50% chance of dying prematurely from a smoking-related illness.*

ABOUT LUNG CANCER

Most of the chest cavity is taken up by the heart and the lungs, with one lung on each side. Air breathed in gets into the lungs through a system of tubes called *bronchi* (Figure 10). The air is eventually distributed into the lung tissue, called *alveoli*, where the gases are exchanged. Breathed-in oxygen passes into our body, and carbon dioxide, the waste product, is removed in the outgoing breath. Cancer-producing agents in tobacco smoke are also inhaled and come into contact with the lining of the bronchi and lung tissue. Some of these cancer-producing substances are absorbed in the lungs, pass into the circulation and can cause cancers elsewhere in the body. Most cancers of the lung originate in the lining of the bronchi, so strictly speaking we should be talking about *'bronchial cancer'*, as only a small proportion originate in the lung tissue itself. However, whether they originate in the bronchi or in the alveoli, by common usage all are called cancers of the lung.

Figure 10: The position of the lungs, bronchi and windpipe (trachea) in the body

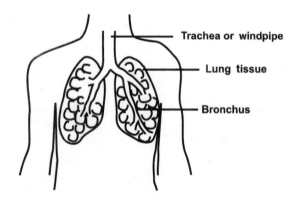

In 1999, over 900,000 instances of lung cancer will be identified around the world, and of these about 180,000 will be in the USA, 37,000 in the United Kingdom, and 9000 in Australia. The outlook for the person who develops lung cancer is much gloomier than that for someone with colorectal cancer, breast cancer or skin cancer, as about nine out of ten people developing lung cancer will die prematurely as a result.

Unfortunately there are no early warning signs that a lung

cancer is developing. The person may feel generally unwell and tired, or they may develop a cough with phlegm or blood in the phlegm. Symptoms such as chest pain, shortness of breath, hoarseness or recurrent chest infections are almost always later symptoms and tend to occur once the lung cancer has become established.

CAUSES OF LUNG CANCER

The causes of lung cancer are shown in Table 16.1. It is clear that most of the blame lies with tobacco use.

Table 16.1: Causes of lung cancer

Smoking causes 85% or 17 of 20 lung cancers

Other than smoking causes 15% or 3 of 20 lung cancers
- Chronic lung disease
- Excessive radiation to the chest
- Workplace or home (Chapters 12 and 13)
  Passive smoking
  Asbestos fibre
  Radon gas
  Other agents
- Inherited tendency
- Dietary habit (Chapter 5)
  Low in vegetables
  High in fat and meat

A PERSONAL RISK LIST FOR LUNG CANCER

If one or more of the situations shown in Table 16.2 is present, there is an increased risk of developing lung cancer. It does *not* mean that lung cancer will develop in the future for certain, since most people classified as having an increased risk do not in fact develop lung cancer during their lifetime. This check list merely means that if the 'yes' column is ticked one or more times, the best advice is to take action which is likely to lower the chances of developing lung cancer.

Table 16.2: Risk factors for lung cancer

Due to lifestyle risks	Yes	No
Tobacco use		
Due to home, environment and workplace risks		
Tobacco smoke—passive smoking (Chapter 13) Asbestos fibre (Chapters 12 & 13) Radon gas (Chapter 12) Other physical and chemical agents (Chapter 12)		
Due to personal health risks		
Family history of lung cancer Chronic lung disease (such as emphysema or lung scarring) Excessive radiation to chest Previous lung cancer removed		

PRIMARY PREVENTION OF LUNG CANCER

Primary prevention is extremely important in lung cancer, because most causes are reasonably easily preventable, and also because screening methods are not well developed nor as effective as in some other cancers, such as in colorectal cancer or skin cancer. The key primary prevention measures are

- **Avoid all forms of tobacco use**
- **Avoid all tobacco smoke**

Other primary prevention methods are summarised in Table 16.3.

Table 16.3: Other than non-smoking, primary prevention measures

- Protect your home, workplace (Chapters 12 & 13)
  Tobacco smoke—passive smoking
  Asbestos fibre
  Radon gas
  Several workplace agents
- Eat plenty of vegetables, fruit and cereals (Chapter 5)

Quitting smoking

In Chapter 6, it has already been described that four out of five smokers find it difficult to quit smoking, partly because smoking is so addictive, partly because of life's stresses, and sometimes because friends or other circumstances in life make it difficult for that person to stop. There is no best way to quit smoking and both complete withdrawal, going 'cold turkey', or gradual cessation of smoking have their problems. Current smokers who are planning to quit could read again the suggestions for a quit smoking programme in Chapter 6 of this book.

Over and above personal measures to quit smoking, it is hoped that as the bad effects of smoking are more widely publicised, companies, large corporations, offices, restaurants, and bars will increasingly make it difficult for anyone to smoke on their premises. Interestingly, major US tobacco companies have finally acknowledged some liability in relation to cigarette smoking. We also hope that our parliaments and regulatory bodies will legislate to ensure increasingly severe restrictions and taxes on smoking and on smokers, so that sometime during the 21st century we become a tobacco-free society, and eventually a tobacco-free world!

EARLY DETECTION OF LUNG CANCER USING SCREENING TESTS

Early warning symptoms of lung cancer are uncommon. However, they include a general feeling of ill-health and tiredness, and sometimes a persistent cough. Sometimes recurring bronchitis or chest infection which is difficult to clear may be present. Even then, these symptoms often occur when the lung cancer is firmly established. Chest x-rays and sputum cytology are sometimes used as screening tests. Bronchoscopy and lung biopsy are methods used for diagnosis rather than for screening.

Screening tests for lung cancer

Unfortunately, there are no satisfactory screening tests for the detection of early lung cancer.

Chest x-ray

X-raying the chest is the simplest means of detecting a lung cancer, by showing a mass in the lungs, although many small lung cancers are not visible on a chest x-ray. Computed tomographic scanning (CAT scan) identifies more lung cancers than a simple chest x-ray.

Sputum cytology

This refers to a method in which sputum (phlegm) is placed under a microscope by a pathologist to detect lung cancer cells which have been shed from the tumour. The test itself is quite accurate when positive, that is, when the pathologist believes that some of the shed cells are cancer cells. The problem is that even regular sputum cytology only picks up well below half of all early lung cancers. However, when regular chest x-rays and sputum cytology are combined, their effectiveness improves. Three out of four lung cancers can be identified by using chest x-ray and sputum cytology together. In the writer's opinion, sputum cytology tends to be underused in the early detection of lung cancer.

Bronchoscopy

This is a diagnostic method used when something suspicious has been shown on a chest x-ray or by sputum cytology. It involves passing a flexible lighted tube down the bronchi, so that the air passages can be seen directly. A biopsy can also be taken of any suspicious area. Cytology can also be performed during bronchoscopy. This involves passing a little saline down the bronchoscope and sucking it back up, then subjecting the fluid, known as *bronchial washings*, to a cytology test.

Biopsy or cytology

There are several ways in which a definite diagnosis of lung cancer can be made. This can be cytology on sputum, biopsy or cytology during bronchoscopy, by passing a fine needle through the skin into the lung and removing a piece of tissue, or during an open operation.

RECOMMENDATIONS FOR SCREENING TESTS

For non-smokers who have no symptoms and no risk factors, screening tests have not been useful and are not recommended. For smokers without any symptoms, anticancer organisations do not recommend mass or population screening with chest x-rays and sputum cytology. Moreover, these tests have not been shown to be cost effective when used for mass screening. However, my personal opinion is that for heavy longstanding smokers (say 40 cigarettes or more per day for over 20 years), when there are other risk factors present, and when such individuals seek screening advice, physician-directed yearly chest x-rays, and yearly sputum cytology starting at age 40 is reasonable, and will identify at least some early and potentially curable lung cancers which would not have otherwise been found (Table 16.4).

Table 16.4: Screening for lung cancer

Non-smokers, no other risk factors, no symptoms
• No screening tests recommended
Heavy smokers and other risks present, no symptoms (only if request screening from medical practitioner)
• Yearly chest x-ray, starting age 40
• Yearly sputum cytology, starting age 40

THE FUTURE FOR LUNG CANCER PREVENTION AND SCREENING

Avoiding all forms of tobacco and tobacco smoke is by far the most important measure in preventing lung cancer. *With increasing public awareness of the dangers of smoking, and with increasing restrictions from regulatory bodies as well as from public and private institutions and other places where people gather, the hope is that a tobacco-free and a smoke-free world will eventuate sometime during the 21st century, thereby lowering the number of individuals who develop lung cancer by 85%. Other primary prevention measures are to remove or protect oneself from physical and chemical agents found at home, in the neighbourhood and in the workplace. Early detection measures using chest x-rays and sputum cytology are of limited value and are probably best restricted to a small subgroup of motivated very high risk individuals.*

17

Prostate cancer

Cancer of the prostate is now the most commonly diagnosed cancer among men. Every year more men are found to have prostate cancer, because it is more common among older men, and men are now living longer, and also because a blood test can now identify a 'silent' or symptomless prostate cancer.

It is difficult to get men to go to a doctor for a cancer check. They seem to experience fear, suspect that a prostate check means they are losing their virility, are often secretive about their health, and quickly dismissive of the suggestion that they could have any health problems.

ABOUT PROSTATE CANCER

It has been estimated that 1 in 10 men, or 10%, will develop prostate cancer during their lifetime. It is estimated that in 1999

Figure 11: The position of the prostate gland in the male pelvis

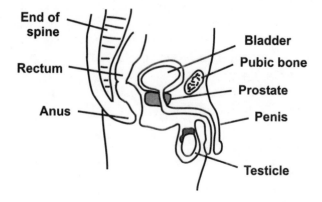

about 300,000 men will be diagnosed with prostate cancer in the USA, about 18,000 in the UK, and 8000 in Australia.

The prostate is a small glandular organ the size of a large walnut, situated at the base of the bladder (Figure 11). It is composed of glandular and fibrous tissue contained in a tough capsule.

The back surface of the prostate can be felt during a digital rectal examination. You may remember that this is a means of examining the last 8–10 cm (3–4 inches) of the rectum as well (Chapter 14). Digital rectal examination is therefore used as a screening test for both lower rectal and prostate tumours.

The outlook in prostate cancer is very good if the cancer is caught early, before it has had a chance to spread outside the capsule of the prostate. The outlook becomes gloomier if the cancer is being treated after it has spread outside the capsule of the prostate and into the tissues of the pelvis, into the local lymph glands, or to distant organs such as the bones.

EARLY SYMPTOMS AND ABNORMAL SIGNS

Cancer of the prostate is often 'silent' and it is uncommon to have early symptoms. Often it grows very slowly and sometimes does not grow at all for several years. Many men die from other causes, and have a small 'silent' prostate cancer, which during life did not cause any symptoms. However, a proportion of prostate cancers are aggressive and can grow quite quickly. Symptoms commence when the prostate cancer presses on the urinary passage or urethra, and causes disturbances of urination such as a poor and weak urinary stream, the need to pass urine frequently, dribbling, or some incontinence of urine. These symptoms also occur when the prostate enlarges due to a form of non-malignant enlargement called benign prostatic enlargement, a condition which is even more common than prostate cancer.

CAUSES OF PROSTATE CANCER

The causes of this cancer are not well known. A hormonal cause fits in with several scientific studies. Men and women each have both male and female sex hormones, although men have a much greater proportion of male sex hormones like testosterone, and women have a greater proportion of female sex hormones like oestrogens. It is held that prostate cancer is related either to an unusually high testosterone level, or a high male-to-female sex hormone proportion. This hormonal imbalance can be caused by a number of factors, which include inheritance, dietary factors or physical inactivity. It has even been found that smoking may increase testosterone levels, or at least increase the male-to-female sex hormone proportions. The factors listed below have been examined by researchers who have linked them with an increased risk for prostate cancer.

- *Inherited predisposition.* A close relative having prostate cancer is an uncommon but important risk, and particularly so if the prostate cancer of the relative had been diagnosed at a relatively early age.
- *Occupational factors.* The use of pesticides among farmers, the use of cadmium among battery or alloy production workers, and the use of chemicals by those doing electroplating are risks.

- *High-fat diet, being overweight or obese, and physical inactivity.* We have seen that a high-fat diet, being overweight or obese and being physically inactive often go together, and it is difficult to separate the contribution of each to the development of a cancer. These aspects of lifestyle increase the chances of developing prostate cancer. With prostate cancer, a high fat diet associated with a low intake of beta-carotene and vitamin E containing foods, and a low intake of cruciferous vegetables and legumes may also be a risk. Inadequate exposure to sunlight (vitamin D), and a low fish intake also seem to be factors which increase a man's chances of developing prostate cancer.
- *Vasectomy.* If vasectomy is done at a relatively young age, it is a possible but unproven risk.
- *Smoking.* This is a possible but unproven risk for prostate cancer.

CHANGES FROM NORMAL CELLS TO CANCER

The changes in prostate cells as they develop from a normal cell to a cancer cell are not as well known as are these changes in some other cancers, such as cancers of the colon or rectum. When prostate tissue is examined by a pathologist under the microscope, there may be cell changes which are in themselves not regarded as an invasive cancer, but which do indicate that the man concerned has an increased chance of developing prostate cancer in the future. These are precancerous changes, and these men need to have a careful follow-up. Such precancerous cells in the prostate are called *prostatic intra-epithelial neoplasia* (PIN).

A PERSONAL RISK LIST FOR PROSTATE CANCER

The check list in Table 17.1 is divided into two, for those who are considered *average risk*, that is, they have no known risk factors and have no symptoms, and for those who are *higher than average risk* because they have one or more risk factors, although they do not have any symptoms. In the presence of urinary symptoms, such as difficulty with the urinary stream, frequent urination during the day or at night, dribbling or incontinence, screening is not appropriate, and a urologist needs to be consulted in order to discover the cause, and commence appropriate treatment. Men with urinary symptoms require precise diagnosis of the cause, and this is outside the scope of this book.

Table 17.1: Risk factors for prostate cancer

	Yes	No
Higher than average risk, no symptoms		
Due to inherited risk • Family member with prostate cancer Due to personal health risk • Previous prostatic biopsy showed *prostatic intra-epithelial neoplasia* (PIN) Due to occupational risk • Pesticide use—farmers • Cadmium exposure—battery or alloy manufacturing and electroplating Due to lifestyle risk • High fat diet • Overweight or obese • Physically inactive		
Average risk, no symptoms		
• Men aged 50 years or more, no symptoms, no risk factors		

PRIMARY PREVENTION OF PROSTATE CANCER

The general principles recommended in a cancer prevention programme for diet (Chapter 5), for smoking (Chapter 6), and for physical activity (Chapter 9), and the precautions which need to be taken among those using pesticides or working with cadmium in industry (Chapter 12), form the basis of primary prevention of prostate cancer. Here, I emphasise what is especially important in the primary prevention of prostate cancer as far as this is known at present. Primary prevention measures are likely to be useful, although they have not been proven to be so beyond doubt. Much research is proceeding currently to determine the role of primary prevention in prostate cancer.

- *Dietary change.* The diet recommended in Chapter 5 is appropriate for the prevention of prostate cancer. Special emphasis is on a very low-fat diet, with fat contributing not more than 20% of the calorie intake. Additionally, it is important to eat plenty of food containing beta-carotene, large quantities of which are contained in carrots, and also in spinach, broccoli, pumpkin, apricots, cantaloup and peaches. Vitamin E containing foods (wheat bran, wheat germ, spinach, sweet potato, peanuts and vegetable oils) are also protective for prostate cancer. A high consumption of all types of fish may be especially useful in the prevention of prostate cancer, possibly through the effects of the omega–3 fatty acids found mainly in fish. Fish is also rich in *selenium*, a trace element, which may also be a protective factor in prostate cancer. Linolenic acid found in linseed can be converted in the body into the essential fatty acids found in fish, and this may also be useful in the dietary prevention of prostate cancer. We get most of our vitamin D from sunlight. However, those who are unable to be in the sunlight or who have particularly dark skin, can obtain vitamin D from eating oily fish. There are, for example, enormous amounts of vitamin D in cod liver oil. A high consumption of cruciferous vegetables (cauliflower, broccoli, cabbage, turnip) may also be a protective factor for prostate cancer.

  Scientists have recently introduced an exciting dimension to the dietary prevention of prostate cancer. They have suggested that eating foods containing oestrogens of vegetable origin (*phytoestrogens*) with lignins and isoflavones such as found in legumes like beans and bean sprouts, soya bean (tofu) and chick peas (homus), may be valuable, particularly in the prevention of prostate cancer. These foods are useful, possibly because they alter the testosterone/oestrogen balance. Recently in Australia, grained breads have been introduced containing both soy and linseed; they are delicious to eat, and may turn out to have beneficial effects in the dietary

178

prevention of prostate cancer and in other conditions such as the relief of menopausal symptoms. Several nutritional supplements made from phytoestrogen-rich legumes especially soy and red clover, have also been produced recently. The value of these supplements in the primary prevention of prostate cancer has not been so far scientifically tested. In this regard also, a compound called *finasteride*, which alters the testosterone/oestrogen balance, is being studied in the USA in the primary prevention of prostate cancer. In another recent study, *vitamin E supplement* was found to decrease the risk of prostate cancer in male smokers by one-third. Selenium supplements may also decrease prostate cancer risk. Based on these recent study results, it would be reasonable for men over 50 years of age, over and above eating an appropriate diet, to also include a daily supplement of 500 units of vitamin E and 200 micrograms of selenium.

- *Smoking.* The smoking connection with prostate cancer has not been established. Nevertheless, smoking is such a hazard for health that it is best avoided anyway (Chapter 6).

- *Physical activity.* In Chapter 9, 30 minutes or more of physical activity on five or more days per week was suggested, exercise in which the pulse rate is raised and there is some sweating. Useful and simple activities include brisk walking, jogging, cycling, swimming or gymnasium work. *It is essential to consult a medical practitioner before commencing a physical activity programme, in order to be pronounced medically fit for such regular physical activity.*

- *Use precautions for occupational hazards* when using pesticides, or if working with cadmium. Please refer to Chapter 12 for more information.

EARLY DETECTION OF PROSTATE CANCER USING SCREENING TESTS

- There are two relatively simple screening tests, *digital rectal examination* and the *prostate specific antigen* (PSA) blood test. At present most public health and anticancer organisations argue against both digital rectal examination and prostate specific antigen tests for population or mass screening of prostate cancer, because on the available evidence there has been no overall benefit. The following discussion relates to men who are motivated to seek screening from their medical practitioner. It is assumed that under these circumstances full screening advice is given to them by their doctor prior to any screening procedure being done.

Other special tests are for diagnosis if symptoms are present, or if there are suspicious findings on digital rectal examination or with the PSA blood test. These diagnostic tests include a *rectal ultrasound examination,* which is often combined with *prostatic needle biopsy.*

Screening tests for prostate cancer

Digital rectal examination

The gloved finger of a medical practitioner is introduced into the rectum, and the back surface of the prostate can be felt for any thickening, swelling or mass. This test may be uncomfortable, but it is never painful and need not cause embarrassment. Public health and anticancer organisations do not recommend this procedure for mass screening. However, on an individual basis it is a harmless procedure, which can lead to the diagnosis of an early and curable prostate cancer.

Prostate specific antigen blood test (PSA)

The glandular cells of the prostate regularly produce a substance called *prostate specific antigen,* which is released into the blood stream and which has a low level in those who have a normal prostate gland. The PSA reading tends to increase slightly with age. The PSA level in the blood stream is often elevated in those who have a prostate cancer. The problem is that men with a benign prostatic enlargement, or with prostate infections, conditions which are completely unrelated to prostate cancer, can also have an elevation of PSA, and this is called a *false positive PSA test for prostate cancer.* Moreover, men who in fact have a prostate cancer can have normal levels of PSA, and this is called a *false negative PSA test for prostate cancer.* It has been estimated that false positive PSA tests occur in about 20% of cases, and similarly false negative PSA tests also occur in about 20% of cases. This means that the PSA test is not informative in 2 of 5 men being screened, and this together with the often slow growth of prostate cancer and the lack of demonstrable benefit in outcome when the entire population is considered, are the reasons why mass screening with PSA has not won support from anticancer organisations.

In spite of its shortcomings, the PSA test can be a useful guide, because an elevation identifies men who may need further investigation, including prostate biopsy. In some of these men, an early and curable prostate cancer is in fact discovered. At present, more than half of all prostate cancers identified by PSA screening in developed countries are confined to the prostate gland, and are therefore curable using currently available treatment. Moreover, this test is also useful in those who may have a slight elevation of their PSA, and a prostate gland that feels normal on digital rectal examination. Urologists usually do not recommend a prostatic biopsy in such situations, but when the PSA is repeated six months or one year later and it shows a further elevation in the interval, a prostatic biopsy is usually recommended. However, if the initial PSA is very high, say six or eight times above the normal value, and if prostatic infection can be excluded, then such a test result usually means that the person does indeed have a prostate cancer.

Diagnostic tests for prostate cancer

Rectal ultrasound and prostatic biopsy

If rectal examination raises suspicions that there may be a prostate cancer, and/or if the PSA reading is elevated or has become progressively elevated between two tests, then a more precise prostate investigation is suggested. At present the most precise means of doing this is to introduce a small ultrasound device into the rectum, and the images obtained from this will guide the surgeon in performing several biopsies in different parts of the prostate gland, using a special needle designed for this purpose, which is inserted into the prostate gland through the rectum. Anaesthetic is not usually necessary. The procedure can cause discomfort and occasionally transient pain. It is usually without side-effects, but sometimes after the procedure there is some transient bleeding with urination. Any transient infection can usually be prevented by the administration of appropriate antibiotics, given at the time of the biopsy.

Needle biopsy

This is a diagnostic test and not a screening test. As with other biopsies using a needle, such as needle biopsy of the breast, the accuracy of this test should be interpreted in the following way. If the result is returned as positive for prostate cancer, this is almost always accurate and we can assume that a prostate cancer is present. If the result is returned as negative for prostate cancer, we cannot be 100% sure that a cancer is *not* present, because sometimes the needle misses the cancer and removes an adjacent piece of non-cancerous tissue. Obviously the earlier and smaller the prostate cancer is, the harder it is for the biopsy needle to hit its target, and therefore biopsies are often taken from several parts of the prostate gland during one procedure.

RECOMMENDATIONS FOR SCREENING TESTS

Only those men who have no symptoms referable to their prostate or bladder are the subjects of the recommendations made in Table 17.2. If symptoms are present, then the cause needs to be diagnosed and these men do not fall into the category of those to be screened for prostate cancer. It is necessary to divide men into two groups, that is, those who have no known risk factors and whom we describe here as 'average risk', and those who have one or more known risk factors. Neither group has any symptoms. Because prostate cancer often grows relatively slowly, it has been found to be of very little value to screen men who are older than 70 years of age. Age 70 is currently regarded as the upper age limit for prostate cancer screening.

Currently, the PSA test is *not* recommended for mass screening. The recommendations which are made in Table 17.2 are directed at men who are motivated and *seek screening*, and an explanation of the pros and cons of PSA testing is given by their medical practitioner before the test is performed.

Table 17.2: Screening for prostate cancer (Only for men who seek screening, and procedure is doctor directed)

No known risk factors, no symptoms, aged 50–70 years
- Annual digital rectal examination
- Annual prostate specific antigen (PSA) blood test

One or more risk factors, no symptoms, aged 45–70 years
- Annual digital rectal examination
- Annual prostate specific antigen blood test (PSA)

THE FUTURE FOR PROSTATE CANCER PREVENTION AND SCREENING
More research is required to understand the causes of prostate cancer. Men need to be motivated through education to pursue primary prevention as far as this is known at present, and in the manner indicated earlier in this chapter. Phytoestrogens in the diet hold out an important hope in dietary prevention. The compound finasteride is undergoing a large scale trial in the USA for the primary prevention of prostate cancer, and the results of this are awaited. Until more accurate screening tests become available, we need to rely on digital rectal examination, and prostate specific antigen (PSA) blood tests for the early detection of prostate cancer. Prostate cancer screening is reasonable provided the men are under 70 years of age, they are motivated and actively seek screening, and provided all screening advice is physician-directed.

18

Malignant melanoma
and other skin cancers

Skin cancers are the most common malignant tumours in developed Western countries. The most common type of skin cancer, *basal cell carcinoma*, spreads only in its vicinity, it never spreads to lymph glands or elsewhere in the body, and is rarely fatal, yet it can cause much disfigurement and unhappiness. The second most common skin cancer is *squamous cell carcinoma*, which spreads locally and sometimes also spreads to the lymph glands or further afield, and is very occasionally fatal. Basal cell and squamous cell cancers are the two important 'non-melanoma' skin cancers. The last is *malignant melanoma*, often simply called *melanoma*. It is a dark, pigmented skin cancer, and if untreated spreads to the local lymph glands and to other distant organs such as the liver, lung and brain. If not treated early, malignant melanoma can be fatal.

Scientific studies in the past two decades have thoroughly confirmed the old belief that excessive sunlight is the most important cause of all skin cancers.

Curiously, whilst scientists are busily sorting out the causes of skin cancer and the best methods of prevention, the scientific advances of some 60 years ago which enabled us to have refrigeration and air conditioning, may inadvertently result in some increase in skin cancer. Chemical compounds, chlorofluorocarbons, used in refrigeration, air conditioning and in other ways, ascend into the atmosphere and deplete the ozone layer which normally filters out most of the harmful ultraviolet rays. There is now an international agreement to decrease and eventually ban the emission of chlorofluorocarbons at the beginning of the next century. This agreement, the widespread concern, and the steps already taken to deal with ozone depletion in many countries, may mean that the predicted harmful effects, which include a large increase in new skin cancers in the 21st century, may not be as dramatic as predicted.

About skin cancer

The skin consists of a superficial layer called the *epidermis*, and a deeper layer called the *dermis*. All skin cancers are found in the superficial layer. Figure 12 shows the microscopic structure of the skin with the most superficial layer of *squamous cells*

Figure 12: Microscopic structure of the skin, showing the cells from which various skin cancers develop, namely squamous cell (squamous cell cancer), basal cell (basal cell cancer), and melanocyte (malignant melanoma)

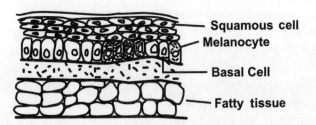

(the origin of squamous cell cancer), beneath which is the *basal cell layer* (the origin of basal cell cancer), and near the basal cells are some pigment cells called *melanocytes*, the origin of malignant melanoma.

Basal cell carcinoma is commonly non-pigmented, and usually begins as a small, often round protuberant pearly swelling. If it remains untreated for a long time it can become an ulcer. It usually grows very slowly and enlarges over a period of months or sometimes years. It is usually treated by surgical excision, occasionally by radiotherapy, or removed by other means.

Squamous cell carcinoma is usually a non-pigmented skin cancer, and it is somewhat more malignant in its behaviour than basal cell carcinoma. The usual appearance of this cancer in the early stages is that of a red, crusty or scaly sore. It often grows more quickly than a basal cell carcinoma. It spreads locally, but this cancer can also spread to the lymph glands and occasionally to distant parts of the body if it remains untreated. The usual treatment for a squamous cell carcinoma is surgical excision.

A *solar keratosis*, sometimes also called a *sunspot,* is a scaly skin thickening, usually brownish or reddish in colour and it usually occurs in response to sun damage. These can turn into a squamous cell carcinoma, and they are also a warning sign that the skin has been sun damaged and is prone to the development of skin cancer.

Malignant melanoma is usually a dark and often irregularly pigmented mark on the skin, flat in its early stages, sometimes with irregular borders. Early malignant melanomas are like unusual freckles—they are flat, pigmented and often have irregular borders and irregular colouring. Melanomas can start from a pigmented mole, or can start in a place where no mole existed previously. A pigmented skin lesion which is changing in appearance is another feature which raises suspicion that it may be a melanoma. If left untreated it usually spreads locally, and if it remains untreated it will spread to the lymph glands and to distant parts of the body such as the liver, brain or lungs. If this condition is untreated or is treated late, it may prove fatal.

The most common form of treatment is surgical excision, and sometimes this is combined with chemotherapy.

It is unknown how common these cancers are globally. However, in the USA alone in 1999, over 500,000 individuals are expected to develop basal cell carcinoma, about 150,000 people are expected to develop squamous cell carcinoma, and about 40,000 individuals are expected to have malignant melanoma. Australia has some of the highest skin cancer rates in the world, and over 150,000 non-melanoma skin cancers and over 6000 melanomas are expected during 1999. It has also been estimated that in Australia, almost half of all men and women will develop a skin cancer of some type during their lifetime.

EARLY SYMPTOMS AND ABNORMAL SIGNS

Basal and squamous cell carcinoma

A persistent, often red or grey skin swelling, nodule or scaly thickening is the early warning symptom or sign. A skin ulcer which does not heal usually indicates a more advanced stage.

Malignant melanoma

The appearance of a new mole, an unusual freckle, or a change in the colour, shape or size of a previous mole or pigmented area of the skin are the early warning symptoms and signs of a melanoma. Early melanomas are usually flat, and may have irregular borders or irregular colouring. Bleeding or ulceration of a mole usually denotes a more advanced stage of the melanoma.

CAUSES OF SKIN CANCER

In this description all skin cancers are included and will only be referred to individually if a particular cause affects only one of the cancers.

- *Excessive sunlight and sunburn especially at a young age.* This is by far the most important single cause of all skin cancers. In Western countries about 9 in 10 of all skin cancers are related to excessive sun exposure. Excessive sunlight during childhood, adolescence or young adulthood is an important risk for all skin cancers, and especially so for malignant melanoma. For all skin cancers the risk level depends not only on the number of episodes of acute sun exposure with sunburn, but also on total lifelong exposure to sunlight, which includes adult life exposure too, such as that experienced by outdoor workers or during outdoor recreational activities.

- *Inherited predisposition.* Those with a fair complexion, whom we would call 'Anglo-Saxon' or 'Celtic', with red or blonde hair, blue or light-coloured eyes, fair skin which does not tan easily but burns easily in the sunlight, with many freckles and moles, are the people whose skin is predisposed to skin cancer. Complexion is inherited, but it is not known whether the tendency to develop skin cancer in these individuals is also inherited. A family history of non-melanoma skin cancer doubles the risk of developing a skin cancer. The more melanocytes there are in the skin, the darker the skin is, and the more the skin is able to tan and not burn, the lower the chances of developing skin cancer. The lowest incidence of skin cancer occurs in black Africans and African-Americans, but no skin is immune to skin cancer, and particularly not malignant melanoma. The chances of developing malignant melanoma are about 40 times greater for white skinned people than for black skinned people.

  A history of malignant melanoma in the family may represent the condition of hereditary melanoma. This forms about 2% of all malignant melanomas. This type of malignant melanoma may be due to an inherited mutation, the CDKN2A gene, as may be the condition described below, the *dysplastic naevus syndrome.*

  Familial dysplastic naevus syndrome (DNS), also called

familial atypical multiple mole melanoma syndrome (FAMMM), is an uncommon inherited condition in which the affected members of the family have 50 or more moles, and are prone to malignant melanoma developing, sometimes in non-sun exposed parts of the body. This condition may be due to an inherited mutation, the CDKN2A gene, although this has not been conclusively established. Research is rapidly heading towards genetic testing using a blood test to identify affected family members.

Xeroderma pigmentosum is a rare inherited condition which predisposes affected family members to various skin tumours.

- *Lowered immune state.* This can occur in individuals who have leukaemia or lymphoma, possibly because of the *immune-suppressing drugs* they are receiving as part of their treatment. Similarly, those with kidney or other transplants can also develop skin cancers when drugs are given to suppress immunity in an attempt to prevent rejection of the grafted organ.

- *Radiation.* Radiographers, radiologists and those receiving industrial radiation, such as in the mining or other industries, may develop skin cancer.

- *Multiple moles, dysplastic moles.* The development of multiple skin moles during life is an important risk for malignant melanomas. This risk increases if microscopic examination of a removed mole contains abnormal or 'dysplastic' cells.

- *Artificial ultraviolet radiation.* This can be obtained from sun-tanning machines or solariums and from home ultraviolet lamps. Possibly also, long-term indoor fluorescent light exposure over many years may be a risk for melanoma, especially on the arms, although this has not been proven beyond doubt.

- *Chronic leg ulcers.* Chronic ulcers of the leg, most of which are associated with varicose veins, can very rarely develop a non-melanoma skin cancer, if the ulcers remain unhealed for many years.

- *Skin cancer from the workplace.* Apart from radiation received in the workplace, those who work with tar, asphalt, pitch, waxes or heavy oils, including shale oil, as well as those who work with arsenic, may develop skin cancer. Farmers and other outdoor workers are prone to skin and lip cancer caused by excessive exposure to the sun.

- *Diet factors.* An undesirable diet low in vitamin A and beta-carotene containing foods, possibly low in vitamin C containing foods, and high in fat is yet another factor which might predispose individuals to skin cancer. Recently it has been found that regular tea drinking may help prevent the development of some skin cancers.

A PERSONAL RISK LIST FOR SKIN CANCER

If one or more 'yes' boxes are ticked in Table 18.1, the person is regarded to be at a higher than average risk for skin cancer. The type of person who is at 'average risk' for skin cancer is shown in Table 18.2.

PRIMARY PREVENTION OF SKIN CANCER

The primary way to prevent skin cancer is to avoid excessive sunlight. Sunscreens are now graded according to their *sun protection factor* (SPF), and their use delays sunburn. It is recommended that for any type of skin SPF15+ needs to be used, and this will screen out over 90% of the sun's rays. It is best to apply the sunscreen before going out in the sun. Apply it again every 2–3 hours while out in the sun, and apply it also after swimming, even for those sunscreens which are said to be water-resistant.

Some public awareness programmes have been enormously successful in altering community behaviour in relation to excessive sun exposure. For example in Australia, the *'Slip Slop Slap'* programme (*Slip* on a shirt, *Slop* on sunscreen, *Slap* on a hat) has resulted in a marked reduction in the total number of sunburns during summertime.

Table 18.1: Risk factors for skin cancer

	Yes	No
Excessive sunlight— evidenced by sunburn episodes with or without blistering, especially during childhood or adolescence Also periods of prolonged exposure to direct sunlight during adult life Artificial ultraviolet rays, such as suntanning machines or home ultraviolet lamps Undesirable diet—a diet high in fat and particularly low in vegetables and fruit of all types is a possible but unproven risk, while tea drinking may be protective		
Due to inherited risk		
Fair complexion with one or more of the following: Does not tan easily, burns easily, red or blonde hair, blue or light eyes, freckles, many moles Family member with melanoma Dysplastic naevus syndrome (DNS), also called familial atypical multiple mole melanoma (FAMMM), xeroderma pigmentosum		
Due to personal health risks		
Previous skin cancer, either non-melanoma or malignant melanoma Previous precancerous conditions removed, such as 'sunspots' (solar keratosis) or 'dysplastic' moles Multiple skin moles Previous skin radiation treatment Previous chemotherapy or immunosuppressant drugs given for leukaemia, lymphoma, kidney or other transplants Longstanding chronic leg ulcer		
Due to occupational risks		
Outdoor workers Exposed to polycylic aromatic hydrocarbons, such as workers in contact with tar, asphalt, heavy oils, waxes, shale oil, automatic lathe workers Industrial radiation, such as radiologists, radiographers, and mining workers		

Table 18.2: Average risk for skin cancer

Average risk person	Yes	No
Men and women 30 years or older for non-melanoma skin cancers, 20 years or older for malignant melanoma, with no risk factors		

Avoid excessive sunlight
- Avoid harsh sun during the middle of the day (from about 11 am to 3 pm). Stay in the shade when outdoors, if possible.
- Cover up whilst in the sunlight.
- Use effective sunscreen on exposed skin.

Avoid artificial ultraviolet radiation
- Avoid suntanning equipment and solariums.
- Avoid home ultraviolet lamps (unless used for the treatment of skin conditions, and done under medical supervision).

Protection against occupational hazards
If employed in one of the industries or professions described below, please read Chapter 12 again for more information on cancer in the workplace.
- Outdoor workers—cover up, use sunscreen.
- Radiation related industries and professions (Chapter 12).
- Those exposed to polycyclic aromatic hydrocarbons (Chapter 12).

EARLY DETECTION OF SKIN CANCERS USING SCREENING TESTS

Almost all skin cancers, including malignant melanomas, are curable if detected early, so that the process of screening for these cancers by inspection alone is simple yet enormously effective.

The screening tests available are quite simple, and these include skin self-examination and a skin check by a medical practitioner.

A further test is a skin biopsy, a diagnostic test used to confirm suspicion of a skin cancer following skin self-examination or a medical skin check. The dramatic advances which have occurred in genetic research are good news for those who may have hereditary melanoma, or are members of families who have *dysplastic naevus syndrome* (DNS), also called *familial atypical multiple mole melanoma syndrome* (FAMMM), because genetic testing using blood tests to identify affected family members is likely to be a practical proposition in the future. The recommendations for the early detection of skin cancers is summarised in Table 18.3.

Screening tests for skin cancer

Skin self-examination

This is simple to perform. All one needs is a full-length mirror, a bright light in the room, and a hand-held mirror for viewing the back of the neck, and parts of the back. It is necessary to look at all parts of the skin including the palms of the hands, soles of the feet, between fingers and toes, under fingernails and toenails, and just inside the mouth lining. Look for pigmented moles, unusual freckles and bumps, or scaly or red sores on the skin. If there are several moles, skin lumps or other suspicious areas, it is best to draw a simple diagram. Attend a medical practitioner for a consultation if there is anything suspicious. If there is any change in previously noted skin moles or freckles, or if new moles or freckles have appeared, also attend a doctor for a check.

Medical skin check

This can be done by a family medical practitioner if experienced in examining the skin for skin cancer, a surgeon, plastic surgeon or a dermatologist. This will be a very complete examination of the skin all over the body.

Skin biopsy

This is usually done with a small injection of local anaesthetic which numbs the skin and then either the whole skin lesion, such as a mole, or a part of it is removed, either with a surgical knife or with what is called a *punch biopsy*, which takes a core of skin only. Very often if surgeons or plastic surgeons are consulted, they will perform an *excisional biopsy* in which the suspicious mole or skin abnormality is completely removed and put under the microscope. The actual biopsy and the subsequent microscopic examination will prove or disprove the presence of a skin cancer conclusively, and also show whether it has been completely removed.

Table 18.3: Recommendations for early detection of skin cancer in women and men

Average risk, no symptoms, 20–49 years
- Skin self-examination 6-monthly

Average risk, no symptoms, 50 years or older
- Skin self-examination 3-monthly
- Medical skin check if there is anything of concern

Higher than average risk, no symptoms, 20 years or older
- Skin self-examination monthly
- Medical skin test yearly, 6-monthly or more often, according to medical advice, if malignant melanoma or non-melanoma skin cancers have been previously removed

THE FUTURE FOR MELANOMA AND SKIN CANCER PREVENTION AND SCREENING

With widespread public education, there is now awareness in many countries, such as the USA and Australia, that if skin cancers are diagnosed and removed early, they are curable with a minimum of inconvenience and often with little or no disfigurement. There is also awareness now that skin cancers can be prevented, principally by the avoidance of exposure to excessive sunlight, and especially so at a young age. Hereditary malignant melanoma is likely to be predictable in the near future with the use of genetic testing. Because of scientific advances in the past which have led to refrigeration and air conditioning, the benefit of which is now reaped not only in developed countries but also in developing and under-developed countries, there may be a depletion of the ozone layer occurring in the stratosphere, so that the harmful rays of the sun are not as well filtered out. Among other important potential problems, such as global warming, this ozone depletion may also result in an increase of all types of skin cancer. We must bring pressure to bear on policy makers and regulatory bodies in developed, developing and under-developed countries to enforce a ban on chlorofluorocarbon emissions by the beginning of the 21st century.

19

Cancer of the cervix

Cancer of the cervix (*cervical cancer*) usually affects women who are younger than those with cancer of the uterus or ovaries. Cervix cancer also has different causes, as well as different means of primary prevention and screening when compared to cancers of the uterus and ovary, and deserves a chapter of its own. Moreover, research into the methods of screening and the primary prevention of this cancer have contributed greatly to our current practices of primary prevention and early detection of cancers elsewhere in the body.

Because of the accessibility of the cervix, and because of a sound knowledge of cervix cancer causes, both primary prevention and screening methods for the early detection of cancer of the cervix are far more advanced than for cancers of the uterus and ovary.

The cervix is the lowest part of the uterus, and its position is shown in Figure 13.

Figure 13: Anatomy of the female reproductive organs, which shows the position of the cervix

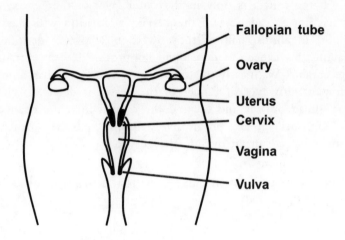

ABOUT CANCER OF THE CERVIX

How common is cervix cancer?

Worldwide, about 500,000 women are expected to develop cervix cancer in 1999, and of these, over 15,000 will be from the USA, about 5000 from the United Kingdom, and over 1000 from Australia.

The outlook for women who develop cancer of the cervix

Overall, the outlook for those women who develop cervix cancer is much brighter than for those who develop cancer of the uterus or ovaries. This brighter outlook is due to the accessibility of the cervix for examination and screening tests, and also because early warning symptoms and abnormal signs in a woman are more frequent with an early cancer of the cervix. We also know more about precancerous stages of cervix cancer, so that we are alert to the possibility of a cancer developing in a woman who has previously had a precancerous condition identified.

If the cancer is only in the outer layer of the cervix, or if it has not spread beyond the cervix, a situation which is now found in almost half of those women who are identified as having this cancer in developed countries, 90% or even more are curable. With early treatment these women can live a normal lifespan. However, if cancer of the cervix is detected when it has spread outside and beyond the cervix, then the chances of a long survival are progressively diminished the further the cancer has advanced outside the cervix.

Precancerous conditions—cervical intraepithelial neoplasia (CIN)

Because of the cervix's relative accessibility, scientists have been able to study precancerous changes directly. These precancerous changes can be detected under the microscope following a cervix smear or biopsy. Cells with an abnormal appearance under the microscope, called *cervical intraepithelial neoplasia* (CIN), represent a precancerous condition. In the earliest cancer stage, localised cancer cells can be seen under the microscope, and this condition can remain dormant and not spread for many years. Interestingly, evidence is accumulating that the precancerous condition of CIN may be reversible in some instances with appropriate forms of primary prevention.

EARLY SYMPTOMS AND ABNORMAL SIGNS

The following are some early warning symptoms or signs.

- Bleeding after intercourse, referred to as *contact bleeding*.
- Spots of blood or obvious bleeding from the vagina.
- A discharge of fluid from the vagina.
- In some women there are no symptoms of any kind.

These early warning symptoms and signs are important to

198

be aware of, as appropriate medical examination will detect an early cancer of the cervix. However, it is emphasised that these symptoms or signs can also be due to non-malignant conditions.

CAUSES OF CERVIX CANCER

The several causes of cancer of the cervix are all related to personal health risks and lifestyle risks. Inherited factors have so far not been identified in this cancer.

Personal health risks

- *Previous sexually transmitted disease (STD)*. Human papilloma virus (HPV) is the most important cause of cervix cancer. Genital herpes (herpes simplex II) is also a risk for cancer of the cervix.
- *Cervical intraepithelial neoplasia (CIN)*. CIN demonstrated on a previous biopsy or smear.
- *Vaginal or vulvar dysplasia*. If for some reason a smear is taken of the vagina or vulva, and this shows dysplasia, it is a risk for cancer of the cervix, as well as for cancer of the vagina.

Lifestyle health risks

- *Early or extensive sexual activity*. This implies sexual intercourse occurring before age fifteen, or pregnancy before age eighteen, or multiple sexual partners and particularly when practising unprotected sexual intercourse, or a history of any form of sexually transmitted disease (STD), or multiple pregnancies, or the use of oral contraceptives started at an early age.
- *Smoking*.
- *Dietary factors*. Undesirable diet as described earlier in Chapter 5 is a contributory factor. Especially for cervix cancer, a low consumption of vegetables and fruit, particularly of the kind containing beta-carotene, vitamin C and folic acid, appears to be a particular dietary risk (Chapter 5). Recent

experimental studies suggest that certain compounds found in raspberries and strawberries confer protection against cancer of the cervix.

A PERSONAL RISK LIST FOR CERVIX CANCER

Higher than average risk for cervix cancer
A woman is at a 'higher than average' risk for cancer of the cervix if one or more 'yes' boxes have been ticked in Table 19.1.

Average risk for cervix cancer
A sexually active woman, 20 years or older, with no risk factors who did not tick any 'yes' boxes in Table 19.1 is regarded to be at 'average risk' for cancer of the cervix.

Table 19.1: Risk factors for cervix cancer

Personal health risks	Yes	No
Previous history of sexually transmitted disease (STD), including human papilloma virus (HPV) and genital herpes		
Previous cervix smear or biopsy showing cervical intraepithelial neoplasia (CIN)		
Previous vaginal or vulval smear or biopsy showing dysplasia		
Personal lifestyle risks		
Early or extensive sexual activity, as gauged by one of the following: sexual intercourse before age 15, pregnancy before age 18, multiple sexual partners, unprotected sexual intercourse, any sexually transmitted disease (STD), multiple pregnancies, oral contraceptives started at an early age		
Smoking		
Undesirable diet (especially one low in vegetables and fruit, and particularly low in beta-carotene, folic acid and vitamin C containing foods)		

PRIMARY PREVENTION OF CERVIX CANCER

For primary prevention of cervix cancer specific recommendations follow.

- *Sexual activity.* Protected sexual intercourse with the male partner using condoms is most important in order to avoid sexually transmitted diseases, including human papilloma virus and genital herpes.
- *Avoid tobacco and tobacco smoke.* Please refer to Chapter 6 regarding the best means of quitting smoking.
- *Dietary changes.* A diet which is particularly high in vegetables, fruit and grains, to include a high consumption of beta-carotene, folic acid and vitamin C containing foods, is important in the dietary prevention of cervix cancer. Please refer to the recommendations made in Chapter 5. As suggested by recent research, the regular consumption of raspberries and strawberries may also protect women against cancer of the cervix. It is most exciting to learn from recent studies that dietary changes have reversed precancerous conditions of the cervix in some women.

EARLY DETECTION OF CERVIX CANCER USING SCREENING TESTS

We can be very optimistic about the early detection of cervix cancer because of the accessibility of the cervix for medical examination, because of the availability of smear tests and biopsies, and also because of our understanding of the evolution of cervix cancer from a normal cell through the precancerous stages to an invasive cancer.

Screening tests for cervix cancer

Medical checkup

This involves a careful history taken by the medical practitioner, as well as a full physical examination, including a vaginal examination, as described below.

Vaginal examination

This is done in the medical practitioner's office or outpatient department of a hospital. It involves the woman being in a prone position, with legs apart. The examination may be uncomfortable and some women may find it embarrassing. However, vaginal examination is usually not painful, especially if the patient is reassured, and if an explanation of what is to be done is provided before the examination. The medical practitioner first examines the outside of the vagina and vulva and then inserts an instrument called a *speculum* into the vagina so that the vagina and mouth of the cervix can be directly inspected for any abnormal thickening, swelling or ulceration. A smear test is then taken. Then a gloved and lubricated finger is inserted into the vagina. Vaginal examination can be complemented by an investigation called *colposcopy,* which is something like a binocular microscope which magnifies the cervix and allows the medical practitioner or gynaecologist to better inspect any suspicious areas in the cervix which may need to be biopsied. This procedure is not painful. Colposcopy is used to better determine the nature of any abnormality found on vaginal examination, and also after an abnormal smear test.

Cervix smear—Pap smear

This test is sometimes called a *Pap smear* after Dr George Papanicolaou, who in the 1920s was the first to suggest that taking a smear around the neck of the cervix and putting the cells under the microscope may be a useful means of diagnosing a precancerous condition or an early stage cancer of the cervix. Although it took almost one generation for this test to be accepted by the medical community, it is now one of the most important cornerstones not only in the early detection of cervix cancer, but also of the precancerous condition of CIN. Moreover, this type of investigation, which has come to be called *cytology*, is most important in the diagnosis and screening of many other cancers and precancerous conditions also. If the cervix or Pap smear is normal and remains normal after successive years, the number of these tests is often decreased and done less often than annually. However, if there is something abnormal or suspicious on the cervix smear, then the test may need to be repeated and often may lead to an actual biopsy of one or several parts of the cervix, a procedure described below. This cervix smear or Pap smear is usually done as part of the vaginal examination, and after the insertion of a speculum. For menstruating women a smear test can be done at any time, except during menstruation. For those who no longer have periods, any time is suitable. The test requires no anaesthetic and does not usually cause pain, although it may cause discomfort or embarrassment.

The cervix or Pap smear test needs to be looked on as a screening test, because in up to 10% of those women who have the test, an early cancer of the cervix or a high grade precancerous condition is present but not identified on the smear. This is called a *false negative test* and in most cases it is due to the smear being taken from a normal part of the cervix. In other instances, abnormal cells are found under the microscope when a cancer of the cervix is in fact not present.

It is important to know that many abnormal cervix smears are not due to cancer. Your doctor will advise the next step if the smear is abnormal.

Recent advances in Pap smear technology include the development of an *automated microscope*, which apparently picks up more abnormal smears than does the conventional method, and a new method of smear preparation, *monolayer technology*, in which the smear can be used once for abnormal cells, and a second time for a *human papilloma virus DNA test*. If the early results are confirmed, the future use of these new methods will make screening for cervix cancer and precancer much more informative and effective.

If someone has had the entire uterus removed previously— *total hysterectomy*—then there is no cervix and usually a smear test is not necessary. It is best to check whether a total hysterectomy has been performed in the past.

Biopsy of the cervix

This test is used for diagnosis, and it is done when the cervix smear is abnormal or suspicious, or when some abnormalities are seen by the medical practitioner in the cervix area during vaginal examination or colposcopy. In the past this procedure was usually performed under general anaesthesia, but now most gynaecologic specialists perform this procedure under local anaesthesia. It can be used for diagnosis, or in those cases in which a cone-shaped biopsy of the circumference of the cervix is made, it can also be used for the treatment of CIN, because the whole area is removed.

RECOMMENDATIONS FOR SCREENING TESTS

For risk factors in cervix cancer, please review Table 19.1 in this chapter.

- *Screening 'average risk' women for cervix cancer with no symptoms.* Two-yearly medical checkup, vaginal examination and cervix smear (Pap smear), starting at age 20, or after sexual intercourse has commenced.

- *Screening 'higher than average risk' women for cervix cancer with no symptoms.* Annual medical checkup, vaginal examination and cervix smear (Pap smear), starting at age 20, or within two years of first sexual intercourse if that occurs before age 20.

THE FUTURE FOR CERVIX CANCER PREVENTION AND SCREENING

Both primary prevention measures and screening tests for cervix cancer are effective. This is because there is a good knowledge of the causes of cervix cancer, because the cervix is accessible for medical examination, smear testing and biopsy, and because smear testing technology is becoming increasingly informative. As a result, death rates from this cancer have decreased but have not been completely eliminated. At least two reasons why prevention and early detection has not been as successful as would be expected is that this cancer frequently occurs at a relatively young age, when the possibility of fatal illness is remote in the thinking of the woman concerned, and also because at that age risk-taking behaviour is common. Creating awareness and motivation for primary prevention and for early detection by screening through education remains an important goal for the future.

20

Cancer of the uterus and ovaries

my womb is round my logic circuitous.
i ache in nervous arcs.
one by one the children come in a curve
out from my pear shaped part.

Excerpt from poem 'Uterus'
Jordie Albiston (1961–)

The female reproductive organs, the uterus or womb, and the ovaries, just like the breasts, are most important for a woman's sense of wholeness and femininity. Cancer of the body of the uterus, *uterine cancer*, cancer of the ovaries, *ovarian cancer*, and cancer of the cervical part of the uterus, *cervix cancer*, are the most common cancers of the female genital organs. Cancers of the vagina and vulva are less common, and cancers arising in the tubes leading from the ovary to the body of the uterus, called the Fallopian tubes, are rare.

In this chapter, uterine and ovarian cancers are described together because their causes, primary prevention and early detection by screening are similar and overlap. Cancer of the cervix, though anatomically part of the uterus, was discussed separately in Chapter 19 because its causes, prevention and early

Figure 14: Anatomy of the female reproductive organs, showing the position of the uterus, cervix, ovaries and Fallopian tubes

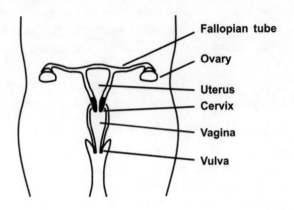

detection by screening tests are different in many aspects from those of uterine and ovarian cancer. The female genital organs are located in the pelvis and the position of the uterus and ovaries is shown in a simplified form in Figure 14.

ABOUT UTERINE AND OVARIAN CANCER

Uterine cancer is diagnosed globally in about 150,000 women each year, and of these, about 35,000 women are in the USA, 5000 in the United Kingdom, and over 1000 in Australia. The outlook for women diagnosed with early uterine cancer is excellent, and three-quarters or more will live out their normal lifespan. When diagnosed late and when the cancer has spread outside the uterus, the long-term outlook is more gloomy.

Ovarian cancer is unfortunately often a highly malignant tumour and it is only uncommonly diagnosed at an early stage. The number of women developing ovarian cancer in 1999 is estimated to be about 170,000 globally, of whom there will be about 27,000 in the USA, whilst in the United Kingdom this figure is 6000 and in Australia 1000. If the ovarian cancer is detected before it has spread from the ovary, the outlook for long-term survival is excellent and there is a 90% chance that the woman will live a normal lifespan. However, if it has spread outside the ovary, which unfortunately currently occurs in 2 out of 3 women who develop this cancer, then the outlook is much more serious, and the chances of long-term survival go down to 25% or less.

Early symptoms and abnormal signs in uterine and ovarian cancer

For *uterine cancer*, abnormal bleeding from the vagina, often in women after the menopause, is the most important symptom and sign. Thus, in the menopausal woman if bleeding recommences, or in the premenopausal woman if there is bleeding between menstrual periods or abnormally heavy bleeding during menstruation, this represents warning signs. About 9 out of 10 women who have uterine cancer will have abnormal vaginal bleeding. However, you should also know that in many instances, abnormal vaginal bleeding is caused not by cancer but by a noncancerous condition, such as fibroids of the uterus.

For *ovarian cancer* there is usually nothing which pinpoints the existence of an early ovarian cancer. Vague discomfort or swelling in the abdomen, sometimes a feeling of nausea, loss of appetite or frequent passage of urine are signs, but these are not specific and can be caused by many other conditions also. The feeling of a lump in the position of the ovary by a medical practitioner is, however, an important sign of a possible ovarian cancer.

Precancerous conditions in uterine and ovarian cancer

Fibroids of the uterus are very common in women. This is a benign condition which almost never becomes malignant. A procedure called *dilatation and curettage* (D&C) in which the lining of the uterus is scraped out in order to identify the cause of any abnormal uterine bleeding, sometimes reveals abnormal tissue showing '*hyperplastic*' or '*dysplastic*' cells under the microscope, and this is a precancerous condition.

Ovarian cysts are very common in women, and these fluid-filled sacs are usually not malignant. If there is a solid part to the lining of these cysts, then they can be precancerous or in fact can be an early cancer of the ovary. *It is emphasised that almost all ovarian cysts which do not have a solid part in their lining are not malignant, and do not predispose a woman to ovarian cancer subsequently.*

CAUSES OF UTERINE AND OVARIAN CANCER

These causes are described together, because they are similar and overlap. In this section, if a cause pertains only to one or the other cancer, this will be indicated. Interestingly, the causes of uterine cancer and ovarian cancer are somewhat similar, or at least overlap with those for breast cancer, described in Chapter 15. These similarities suggest to scientists that female sex hormones may play a part in the development of these cancers, just as they do in the development of breast cancer.

Inherited uterine or ovarian cancer

- *Hereditary non-polyposis colorectal cancer (HNPCC).* In the inherited condition known as hereditary non-polyposis colorectal cancer (HNPCC), sometimes also called Lynch syndrome, women are predisposed not only to colorectal cancer but also to uterine cancer, and to a lesser extent also to ovarian cancer (Chapter 14). A group of mutated genes called MSH2, MLH1, PMS1 and PMS2 appear to be involved.
- *Breast-ovarian cancer syndrome (BOCS).* The mutated gene BRCA1 appears to be involved in this uncommon condition in which both breast cancer and ovarian cancer develops.

Personal health risks

- *Previous breast, colorectal, ovarian or uterine cancer.* The risk of uterine or ovarian cancer is doubled.

- *Hormone replacement therapy with the exclusive use of oestrogen.* This causes a slight increase in risk for uterine cancer, but probably not for ovarian cancer. More recent preparations which contain both oestrogen and progestogens probably do not predispose women to uterine cancer. It is interesting that the use of oral contraceptives actually decreases the chances of a woman developing uterine or ovarian cancer.
- *Polycystic ovary syndrome.* These are relatively uncommon conditions in which women have many cysts in both ovaries.
- *Fertility drugs.* These drugs possibly increase ovarian cancer risk.
- *Tamoxifen use* (in the treatment of breast cancer). Tamoxifen possibly increases uterine cancer risk.
- *A long menstrual life.* By this is meant menstruation beginning early in life before the age of 12, and/or a late menopause, that is, after the age of 50.
- *No children.*
- *High blood pressure or diabetes.*

Lifestyle risks

- *Undesirable diet.* This includes a high-calorie, high-fat, low-vegetable, low-fruit diet, and probably a diet which is also low in fish. A high consumption of legumes, such as beans, appears to confer protection against uterine cancer.
- *Overweight or obese women.* They have an increased chance of developing uterine cancer, and possibly also ovarian cancer.
- *A sedentary inactive life.* This often goes with being overweight or obese, as well as with an undesirable dietary habit as described above.
- *Women who have never used oral contraceptives.* These women are more prone to both uterine and ovarian cancer, suggesting that for reasons which are at present uncertain, the use of oral contraceptives protects women from these two cancers.

A PERSONAL RISK LIST FOR UTERINE AND OVARIAN CANCER

A woman is at a 'higher than average risk' for a cancer of the uterus or ovary if one or more 'yes' boxes have been ticked in Table 20.1.

Women aged 50 or older, with no risk factors who did not tick any 'yes' boxes in Table 20.1, are regarded to be at 'average risk' for cancer of the uterus and ovary.

Table 20.1: Risk factors for uterine and ovarian cancer

Inherited cancer risk	Yes	No
Hereditary non-polyposis colorectal cancer (HNPCC), sometimes called Lynch syndrome Family history of breast-ovarian cancer syndrome (BOCS)—this is a risk for ovarian cancer, not uterine cancer Family history of ovarian cancer		
Personal health risks		
Previous breast, or colorectal, or uterine, or ovarian cancer Previous uterine dysplasia on biopsy of the uterine lining after dilatation and curettage (D&C), or uterine aspiration biopsy Long menstrual life (menstruation commencing before age 12 and/or menopause after 50 years of age) No children Polycystic ovary syndrome History of high blood pressure or diabetes Previous use of fertility drugs (ovarian cancer) or tamoxifen (uterine cancer)		
Personal lifestyle risks		
Undesirable diet (especially high energy, high fat, low vegetable and fruit, and low fish diet) Overweight or obese Physically inactive, sedentary person		

PRIMARY PREVENTION OF UTERINE AND OVARIAN CANCER

> *Since there are no satisfactory screening tests for the early detection of either uterine cancer or ovarian cancer, primary prevention becomes very important.*

- *Dietary recommendations.* Over and above the dietary recommendations in Chapter 5, it is especially important to eat a low-calorie diet which is low in fat and sugar, high in vegetables and fruit, especially foods containing beta-carotene, vitamin C and folic acid, as well as a high fish consumption (Chapter 5). A high consumption of legumes, such as beans, chick peas and soy, has recently been shown to confer some protection against uterine cancer.
- *Weight control.* Overcoming obesity is an important special recommendation for both uterine and ovarian cancer.
- *Physical activity.* This is an important recommendation for both uterine and ovarian cancer. Performing 30 or more minutes of moderate physical activity five or more days each week is recommended. This is exercise which will raise the pulse or induce some sweating, such as brisk walking, jogging, cycling, swimming or gymnasium work. *Before this recommendation to commence regular physical activity is acted upon, it is important to check with a medical practitioner that such a physical programme is compatible with one's general health.*

EARLY DETECTION OF UTERINE AND OVARIAN CANCER USING SCREENING TESTS

The problem with uterine and ovarian cancer is that there are no simple or effective screening tests available. However, there are certain tests that can be performed which may improve a woman's chances of identifying an early uterine or ovarian cancer, particularly if she is at higher than average risk. A medical checkup when combined with a pelvic/vaginal examination can identify a few early and curable cancers of the uterus and ovaries.

Screening tests

A medical checkup

This involves an examination by a medical practitioner, which would include a thorough medical history of past and current health, and a family history of illnesses, including cancer. This would be followed by a thorough physical examination, a vaginal examination described below.

Pelvic/vaginal examination

This is performed in the medical practitioner's office, or in the outpatient department of a hospital. It is uncomfortable and some women feel embarrassed and fearful. However, it usually does not cause pain, and especially not if a reassuring explanation of what is to be done is given before the examination. The vulva is inspected and an instrument, called a *speculum*, is then inserted into the vagina so that the entire vagina and cervix can be inspected. A gloved and lubricated finger is then introduced into the vagina, in order to feel the vagina and the position of the ovaries. The examining doctor also feels the uterus by placing the other hand on the lower abdominal wall. Usually a cervix smear is taken and sometimes a uterine aspiration biopsy is also performed. *This examination can be uncomfortable and embarrassing for some women; however, it can provide a lot of important information regarding the state of the vulva, vagina, cervix, uterus and ovaries.*

Diagnostic tests

Uterine aspiration biopsy

This is usually performed only in women who are at a higher than normal risk for uterine cancer. In this test a fine tube is inserted through the vagina into the cavity of the uterus during pelvic/vaginal examination, and some tissue and fluid is collected by suction from the uterus and its lining. This procedure can be performed in the medical practitioner's office and requires no anaesthetic.

Dilatation and curettage (D&C)

Sometimes more extensive testing of the uterine lining is necessary. A procedure called dilatation and curettage (D&C) may need to be performed, and this is done under a general anaesthetic. In this investigation the entire lining of the uterus is removed with a special instrument, and the tissue so obtained is subjected to examination under the microscope.

Hysteroscopy

This relatively recent test is performed in the doctor's office. An endoscope, which is an optical instrument, is inserted into the uterus, so that its lining can be inspected and any suspicious areas removed for biopsy. At present it is a diagnostic test only, since the cost of the investigation prohibits its use as a screening test.

CA125 antigen blood test

This is a relatively recently developed blood test which is used for the detection of ovarian cancer only. Unfortunately, only about half of all women with early ovarian cancer will have an elevation of the CA125 level above normal. This test is at present more useful to gauge the response of a woman who has had ovarian cancer treated, in order to assess whether there is any evidence of recurrence of this cancer, than it is for screening.

Vaginal/pelvic ultrasound

This is of some value if there is a suspicion of an ovarian cancer. Ultrasound performed in this way, with the detecting device inserted into the vagina for a vaginal ultrasound, and over the lower abdomen for a pelvic ultrasound, can detect early ovarian cancer. The problem is that it also detects other non-malignant conditions of the ovary, such as cysts. An abnormal ultrasound finding may therefore lead to surgery in which an ovarian cancer is, in fact, not found. Ultrasound can also be used to examine the thickness of the uterus lining. In the future this test may be used for screening, to identify women who have an abnormally thick uterine lining, which may be caused by a precancerous condition or an early cancer of the uterus. In such a case, the woman would require further diagnostic tests, and especially a biopsy.

Computed tomographic scan of the pelvis

In this test an abnormal enlargement or swelling, of either the ovary or uterus, can be detected.

Laparoscopy or laparotomy

These are surgical procedures, laparoscopy being a smaller operation than laparotomy. Both are performed under general anaesthesia. In both procedures abnormal enlargements of the ovary or uterus can be detected by direct inspection, and in laparotomy by feeling the organs also. Pieces of tissue can also be removed for biopsy.

RECOMMENDATIONS FOR SCREENING TESTS

Screening average risk women for uterine or ovarian cancer with no symptoms

Annual medical checkup, including pelvic/vaginal examination, is recommended beginning at age 50. Note that in practice medical checkups and pelvic examinations are often performed in conjunction with examinations for the early detection of cervix cancer, so that these examinations would usually commence at age 20 or after the commencement of sexual activity (Chapter 19).

Screening higher than average risk women for uterine or ovarian cancer with no symptoms

Annual medical checkup including pelvic/vaginal examination beginning at age 40. Again, note that in practice these medical checkups are often combined with checkups for the early detection of cervix cancer; therefore a cervix smear is also performed. Checks for cervix cancer usually commence at age 20 (Chapter 19).

> *THE FUTURE FOR UTERINE AND OVARIAN CANCER PREVENTION AND SCREENING*
> *In contrast to cancer of the cervix, which medical science is well on the way to preventing or at least detecting at an early and curable stage, we are still expecting future research into cancers of the uterus and ovaries to discover more precise ways of primary prevention and early detection. Effective screening for these two cancers is not well developed at present.*

21

Stomach cancer

One of the most important consequences of our being animals is that we have got this bottomless pit called the stomach.

The Importance of Living
Lin Yutang (1895–1976)

The stomach is a bag-like organ that forms the upper part of the gut and is the continuation of the oesophagus or gullet. It is an important organ of digestion, and a signaller of hunger. The stomach is situated just under the diaphragm, as may be seen in Figure 15. In common parlance the entire abdomen is sometimes referred to as the 'stomach', although in the medical context the word refers only to the digestive organ situated between the oesophagus and the duodenum, as shown in Figure 15. The medical term for stomach cancer is *gastric cancer*.

ABOUT STOMACH CANCER

How common is stomach cancer?

Earlier this century cancer of the stomach was one of the most common cancers in Western countries, but the number of such

Figure 15: The position of the stomach in the abdominal cavity

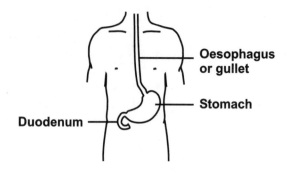

Oesophagus
or gullet

Stomach

Duodenum

cancers has gradually decreased over the past 50 years. This decrease is attributed to refrigeration becoming more easily available, allowing foods to be preserved fresh in a refrigerator rather than being smoked, salted, pickled or cured. These methods of preserving and treating food are believed to be some of the causes of stomach cancer. The rate of stomach cancer is still high in some countries such as Japan and China, regarded as largely due to the dietary habits in these countries, as well as to a high cigarette smoking rate.

Globally, about 800,000 individuals are expected to develop stomach cancer in 1999, and of these, there will be only about 23,000 in the USA, about 12,000 in the United Kingdom, some 1800 in Australia, but some 85,000 in Japan, and over 260,000 in China.

The outlook for stomach cancer

If the cancer can be identified at a time when it only involves the superficial lining layer of the stomach and only involves a few cells, and such a stomach cancer is surgically removed, 90% of these individuals are likely to have a normal lifespan. However, if the stomach cancer has involved all the layers of the stomach, this chance decreases to 50%, and if it has spread outside the stomach or to distant organs of the body, the chances of surviving in the long term are extremely gloomy.

Precancerous conditions in stomach cancer

- *Benign stomach (gastric) ulcer.* In most instances these benign ulcers situated in the stomach do not become malignant, although in a few, cancerous change can supervene after many years. *Helicobacter pylori* infection of the stomach appears to be an important cause of gastric ulcers.
- *Chronic duodenal ulcer.* This is a common condition of the duodenum, the organ situated next to the stomach (Figure 15). We can reassure those with this condition that even after many years of having a chronic duodenal ulcer, the chances of it becoming malignant are almost nil.
- *Gastritis with low or absent stomach acid production.* This situation can occur in an uncommon illness, *pernicious anaemia*, and it can also occur without any obvious reason. Here, absent or low levels of stomach acid which is normally produced to aid digestion, is associated with the disappearance of gastric glands, and this is called *atrophic gastritis*. Atrophic gastritis is a premalignant condition.

CAUSES OF STOMACH CANCER

Inherited causes

- *Family history of stomach cancer.* Such a history in a near relative doubles a person's chances of developing stomach cancer during their lifetime.
- *Type A blood group.* The common blood groups are A, B, O and AB. A person with Type A blood has a 20% increased chance of developing stomach cancer during their lifetime compared to those with other blood groups.

Personal health risks

- *Presence of Helicobacter pylori in the stomach.* This is an organism which in recent years has been associated not only with stomach cancer but also with gastric and duodenal ulcers, and with inflammatory changes called gastritis. Why

Helicobacter infection is present in some individuals but not in others is at present uncertain, although it may be linked to both undesirable dietary habits and to tobacco use. In itself, *Helicobacter* infection probably causes no symptoms. *Helicobacter pylori* infection can usually be eradicated by the use of suitable antibiotics. It has also been suggested recently by Australian scientists that the regular intake of acidophilus bacteria (found in some brands of yoghurt and in some dietary supplements), can also eradicate *Helicobacter* infection.

- *Previous surgical removal of part of the stomach (partial gastrectomy) for a non-malignant condition, such as a gastric or duodenal ulcer.* This becomes a stomach cancer risk some 15–40 years after the stomach has been removed.

- *Pernicious anaemia.* Individuals with this uncommon condition not only have anaemia but also have no normal stomach acid production. They develop the condition previously described, atrophic gastritis. Individuals with atrophic gastritis have a 10% chance of developing stomach cancer during their lifetime.

- *Low or absent stomach acid production with atrophic gastritis.* Even in the absence of pernicious anaemia, this is a risk for the future development of stomach cancer.

Lifestyle health risks

- *Dietary factors.* A special risk for stomach cancer is a diet which is low in vegetables, fruit and cereals, and particularly those fruits, vegetables and cereals which contain a lot of beta-carotene, vitamin C and vitamin E. A diet high in pickled, smoked, salted or cured foods, or foods preserved with nitrate, such as salami, sausages, hot dogs, smoked meat, smoked fish or pickled food of any kind are also risks for stomach cancer. These dietary factors are probably important because the risk foods described above all seem to produce carcinogens called *nitrosamines*. Also, vitamin C acts as an antioxidant and has other actions which neutralise the effects of nitrosamines. Dietary factors are probably the most important single cause of stomach cancer.

- *Smoking*. A recent Australian study which examined all the scientific evidence published over the years has found that smoking is likely to be an important contributory cause of stomach cancer.

A PERSONAL RISK LIST FOR STOMACH CANCER

A 'higher than average risk' is present for stomach cancer if one or more 'yes' boxes have been ticked in Table 21.1.

A person 55 years or older, with no risk factors who did not tick any 'yes' boxes in Table 21.1, is regarded to be at 'average risk' for cancer of the stomach.

Table 21.1 Risk factors for stomach cancer

Inherited risk factors	Yes	No
Stomach cancer in a relative Type A blood group		
Personal health risks		
Helicobacter pylori previously identified in the stomach Previous surgical removal of part of the stomach (partial gastrectomy) for a non-malignant condition of the stomach or duodenum Previously identified pernicious anaemia Low or absent stomach acid or 'atrophic gastritis' identified previously		
Personal lifestyle risk		
Undesirable diet, especially one low in fruit, vegetables and cereals, and high in pickled, smoked, salted or cured foods, or high in foods containing nitrate as a preservative Smoking		

PRIMARY PREVENTION OF STOMACH CANCER

Specific recommendations for primary prevention of stomach cancer

- *Dietary changes*. It is particularly important to have a high consumption of fruit, vegetables and cereals which contain beta-carotene, vitamin C and vitamin E, and at the same time avoid or eat very little pickled, smoked, salted, cured and nitrate-preserved foods (Chapter 5). In a recently reported study from China, where stomach cancer is still relatively common, the daily use of vitamin E, beta-carotene and selenium supplements decreased stomach cancer risk by one-fifth.

- *Avoid smoking*. Hints and guidance about quitting smoking are described in detail in Chapter 6.
- *Eradicate Helicobacter pylori*. If *Helicobacter* infection has been shown to be present, suitable antibiotics can be used. Recent research suggests that the acidophilus bacteria found in some yoghurts and in some dietary supplements may also be an effective way to eliminate *Helicobacter* infection.
- *Aspirin*. Based mainly on experimental data, the regular use of aspirin as a preventive for stomach cancer has been advanced. However, the human evidence of a preventive role for aspirin in stomach cancer is insufficient at present to make such a recommendation.

EARLY DETECTION OF STOMACH CANCER USING SCREENING TESTS

Screening tests—upper gastrointestinal endoscopy

The only useful and effective screening test for the early detection of stomach cancer is to pass a flexible lighted tube through the oesophagus (gullet) and into the stomach to allow direct viewing of this organ. It is also possible during this procedure to remove a small piece of any suspicious area for biopsy. This is a commonly used diagnostic test for inflammation, ulcers or cancer in the oesophagus (gullet), stomach or duodenum.

Upper gastrointestinal tract endoscopy has been used as a screening test but only in countries in which the rate of stomach cancer is very high. This was done successfully in Japan where many early and curable stomach cancers have been identified by this method. This screening test has not been used routinely in countries in which the rate of stomach cancer is relatively low, such as in the USA, UK, Australia or New Zealand, because if used systematically the cost to the community would be enormous, and it would only identify a few instances of early stomach cancer.

Recommendations for the early detection of stomach cancer using upper gastrointestinal endoscopy

Because there is such a large variation in the number of stomach cancers found in different populations around the world, the recommendations for doing upper gastrointestinal endoscopy as a screening test are different in a 'low risk country' such as the USA, Australia or New Zealand, compared to the recommendations for a 'high risk country' such as Japan or China. Although endoscopy is a reasonably safe test which is often done without an anaesthetic, requiring only a simple sedative injection, it uses a lot of resources, and it is expensive. This test therefore cannot be performed routinely in those countries in which there is a low rate of stomach cancer, as in most individuals an actual stomach cancer will not be found.

- *Average risk individuals, 'low risk country', no symptoms.* Upper gastrointestinal tract endoscopy is not recommended.
- *Average risk individuals, 'high risk country', no symptoms.* Endoscopy 1–2-yearly at age 55 or over is recommended. This recommendation may not be feasible for mass screening in most high risk countries for economic reasons and lack of medical resources.
- *Higher than average risk individuals, 'low risk country', no symptoms.* Most anticancer agencies in these countries do not recommend screening tests. However, if several risks are present, and the person seeks screening, a reasonable recommendation would be to perform a baseline upper

gastrointestinal tract endoscopy at age 55 and then, according to the findings, do this 1- or 2-yearly subsequently.

- *Higher than average risk individuals, 'high risk country', no symptoms.* Baseline upper gastrointestinal tract endoscopy is recommended at age 50 and then, according to the findings, further endoscopy every 1–2 years. At a population level this recommendation may not be feasible for cost reasons and lack of medical resources.

THE FUTURE FOR STOMACH CANCER PREVENTION AND SCREENING

It is heartening to see that the number of stomach cancers identified in developed Western countries is gradually decreasing. Primary prevention with a diet in which there is a high intake of foods containing vitamin C, and the avoidance or the infrequent consumption of smoked, salted, pickled or preserved food or nitrate-containing food, as well as the avoidance of tobacco, will ensure that stomach cancer will occur infrequently in the future. It is also hoped that these lifestyle changes will diminish the number of stomach cancers in countries in which it is still prevalent, such as Japan, Korea and China. This means that screening in these countries using expensive upper gastrointestinal tract endoscopy will not often be required in the future.

22

Prevention and early detection of less common cancers

> *Cancer of the anus, bladder, brain, gallbladder, kidney, liver, mouth and throat, oesophagus, pancreas, penis, testicle, thyroid, vagina and vulva, leukaemias, lymphomas and sarcomas*

The prevention and early detection of cancers and other malignant tumours which are not commonly encountered are described here, as are those cancers in which the causes and therefore primary prevention is not well understood, as well as malignant tumours in which screening tests used for early detection are either not available or are not very effective.

Space does not allow a full description of every cancer or malignant tumour, so in this chapter a summary of the main aspects concerning the primary prevention and screening of the cancers not described so far is provided. The extremely uncommon or rare malignant tumours are not described in this book. The various malignant tumours are described in alphabetical order for easy reference, and there is a uniform sequence in which each cancer is presented.

The Introduction briefly describes where the cancer is in the body, how common it is, what the outlook is if an individual develops this cancer, and whether there are any precancerous conditions. Important *early* symptoms or signs of the cancer will be described. A full list of all the symptoms and abnormal signs of that cancer will not be discussed, since this is in the domain of cancer diagnosis rather than cancer prevention and early detection, and is therefore outside the scope of this book.

The section on personal risk summarises the important information of those at an increased risk for this particular cancer. Inherited causes, occupational health risks, personal health risks and personal lifestyle risks is the sequence in which the risk list is described. As far as this is possible, the importance of the risk is 'weighted' by describing it as a 'possible', 'probable' or a 'very likely' risk. If the risk is proven, no weighting is given.

Specific recommendations in the primary prevention of the particular cancer are briefly presented and the available screening tests and recommendations for screening are given.

ANAL CANCER

The anus is the lowest part of the large bowel, and follows the rectum. It commences as the anal canal which is about 2 cm long, and it terminates as the anal orifice, an opening which is visible to the exterior.

Anal cancer is uncommon. It usually grows relatively slowly, and if the cancer is identified early it can usually be removed surgically or treated by radiotherapy and chemotherapy, with a very good outlook and a normal lifespan. Although the cancer is usually visible even in its early stages, it is often neglected by the individual. Precancerous conditions are the *human papilloma virus, warts* around the anus, and the *herpes simplex II virus,* or *genital herpes.*

Early warning symptoms or signs of anal cancer

The following symptoms or signs, all of which can be either seen or felt around the anus, are important early symptoms and signs, and demand medical examination: persistent rash or irritation, discharge, a swelling, thickening or lump, non-healing ulcer, bleeding, or uncommon pain.

It is emphasised that all these symptoms or signs are in fact usually due to non-malignant conditions such as haemorrhoids, fissures or dermatitis, and none are specific to anal cancer. However, when any of these symptoms occur, an early medical checkup is recommended.

A personal risk list for anal cancer

- *Inherited anal cancer.* Inherited factors have not been identified in this cancer.
- *Personal health risks.* Previous history of sexually transmitted disease, human papilloma virus (HPV), anal or genital warts, genital herpes (herpes simplex II), chronic anal conditions, such as fissures and fistulas, use of immunosuppressive drugs.
- *Personal lifestyle risks.* Anal receptive intercourse, male homosexuality, possibly smoking.

Specific recommendations for primary prevention of anal cancer

- Protection with a condom during sexual intercourse (Chapter 10).
- Avoid tobacco use (Chapter 6).

Early detection of anal cancer using screening tests

- *Screening tests available.* A medical checkup which includes inspection and digital rectal examination of the anal area, anal canal and rectum. Any suspicious swelling or thickening, or any warts or lumps at or near the anus or in the anal canal can be removed in part or completely, and subjected to a microscopic examination.

- *Screening recommendations for anal cancer.* Annual general medical check including digital rectal examination commencing at age 50 for all who are at an increased risk for developing this cancer, as gauged from the personal risk list.

BLADDER CANCER

The urinary bladder is located in the pelvis, as shown in Figure 16, and receives the urine produced by the kidneys. In 1999 about 250,000 men and women are expected to be diagnosed with this cancer globally, over 50,000 in the USA, about 13,000 in the United Kingdom, and about 2500 in Australia. If it is diagnosed early, the long-term outlook for this cancer is usually very good, and the cancer can usually be removed without having to remove the bladder itself. However, if the symptoms are neglected and the cancer is identified at a late stage, then the bladder may also need to be removed and the urinary stream diverted. In advanced bladder cancer the eventual outlook is frequently serious. The most important precancerous condition for bladder cancer is a *bladder papilloma*, which is a benign tumour. Bladder papillomas frequently recur after surgical removal.

Figure 16: The position of the urinary bladder in the pelvis

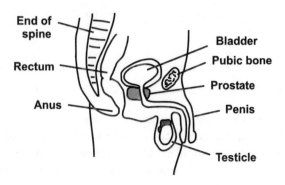

Early warning symptoms or signs for bladder cancer

Most bladder papillomas and 4 out of 5 early bladder cancers will have the symptom of blood in the urine, and/or frequent urination, pain on urination or urgency of urination. Urgency of urination means that the individual has an urgent need to pass urine, they pass it frequently, and often do not pass large quantities at any one time. Persistent symptoms of bladder irritation or blood in the urine require medical attention and usually also referral to a urological specialist. About 1 individual in 5 who develops bladder cancer may not have early warning symptoms or signs.

A personal risk list for bladder cancer

- *Inherited bladder cancer.* None identified.
- *Personal health risks.* Bladder papilloma or bladder cancer previously removed, recurrent bladder infections, previous history of radiation to the pelvis.
- *Occupational health risks.* Chemicals used among dyestuff workers, dye users, workers in aromatic amine manufacturing industries, textile workers, rubber and leather workers, painters, hairdressers, printers, long-term truck, bus and taxi drivers, and aluminium workers.
- *Personal lifestyle risks.* Smoking is an important risk. Excessive past use of pain-relieving medications containing phenacetin (now withdrawn from the market), possibly excessive use of artificial sweeteners, and possibly excessive coffee drinking.

Specific recommendations for primary prevention of bladder cancer

- Avoid smoking (Chapter 6), avoid excessive use of artificial sweeteners and probably also excessive coffee drinking. For occupational exposures, use protection policies described in Chapter 12.

Early detection of bladder cancer using screening tests

- *Screening tests available.* There are no simple screening tests available for bladder cancer. Persistent bladder symptoms such as bleeding, frequent urination or urgency of urination require an examination by a urological specialist, who will usually perform a procedure called *cystoscopy*. In this procedure, a fiberoptic telescope is introduced into the bladder in order to examine the bladder lining and detect any swelling, thickening, inflammation, ulcer formation or a lump which may be a bladder tumour. Any suspicious area can be biopsied and the tissue examined under the microscope. Cystoscopy and biopsy is the definitive means of identifying a bladder papilloma or a bladder cancer.
- *Screening recommendations for bladder cancer.* There are no specific recommendations. Persistent symptoms suggesting an abnormal bladder condition require an early examination by a urological specialist.

BRAIN TUMOURS

Brain tumours are not common in adults. They are, however, one of the major childhood cancers. The two common types are called *gliomas* and *meningiomas*. Gliomas are often very rapid and aggressive in their growth. Meningiomas are usually slow growing and many years can elapse before they cause symptoms. By far the most common malignant tumours in the brain are secondary or metastatic cancers which have spread from another site, with the primary cancer commonly in the lung, breast, bowel or prostate. These secondary brain cancers will not be considered in this section.

Brain tumours are not common, but are increasingly diagnosed. Their increased numbers may in part be due to newer diagnostic tests that are better able to identify these tumours, and in part to new cancer-producing agents. During 1999 it is expected that about 18,000 individuals will develop brain tumours in the USA, about 3500 in the United Kingdom, and about 1000 Australian children and adults are expected to develop this cancer.

Early warning symptoms or signs of brain cancer

There are often no early symptoms or signs. Persistent headache, nausea, vomiting, personality changes and a general slowing in brain function may be due to a brain tumour. An early medical examination, and sometimes an examination by a neurologist or neurosurgeon may also need to be undertaken.

A personal risk list for brain cancer

Unfortunately the causes of brain tumours are not well understood and many who develop brain tumours do not appear to have been exposed to any known risk factors.

- *Inherited brain cancer.* A rare inherited condition called *neurofibromatosis,* which gives rise to swellings under the skin and brown skin patches, can also cause brain tumours. Very occasionally, brain tumours run in families. The mutated genes NF1 and NF2 appear to be involved.
- *Occupational health risks.* Some chemicals used in pesticides and insecticides may be the cause of some tumours in farmers, petrochemical and vinyl chloride industry workers, and rubber workers. Exposure to electromagnetic fields (EMF) may be the cause in electrical and electronic workers. Radiation may be a cause in radiologists, radiographers and uranium miners.
- *Personal health risks.* Past history of head injuries slightly increases the risk of developing a meningioma. Previous radiation, either used as treatment or for diagnosis, such as repeated full dental films, increases the risk of a meningioma and possibly of glioma.
- *Personal lifestyle risks.* An increased consumption of nitrate-containing food found in preserved meat such as sausages

and salami, which in turn leads to the formation of carcinogenic *nitrosamines,* increases the risk of developing a brain
tumour. It is not known whether tobacco smoke which
contains nitrosamines poses an increased risk. Living or
playing near high tension electricity wires may increase the
risk for brain tumours in children, and this is possibly caused
by low frequency electromagnetic fields (EMF) created by
these wires. However, more research is required to substan-
tiate the suggestions that exposure to EMF increases brain
tumour risk.

Specific recommendations for primary prevention of brain tumours

* Avoid or minimise exposure to radiation and electromagnetic fields.
* Use all the necessary protection in the several at-risk occupational exposures.
* Limit intake of nitrate-containing foods.

Early detection of brain tumours using screening tests

* *Screening tests available.* There are no simple screening tests
  available. All the tests are sophisticated radiological investigations used for diagnosis, such as computed tomographic
  scanning and magnetic resonance imaging of the brain.
* *Screening recommendations for brain tumours.* No specific screening recommendations can be made at present. Persistent
  headache, particularly if associated with nausea and vomiting, or with personality changes noticed by family and
  friends, or a general slowing of brain function, demand early
  consultation with a neurologist or neurosurgeon who will
  institute appropriate investigations.

Gallbladder cancer

The gallbladder sits under the liver; it concentrates bile produced by the liver, and this assists with the digestion of food. Its surgical removal—*cholecystectomy*—is compatible with a normal life. Gallbladder cancer is uncommon in Western populations and is more often seen in women than in men. High rates are present in Latin America and among American Indians. Unfortunately the majority of gallbladder cancers are detected at an advanced stage. Most gallbladder cancers appear to be causally linked to pre-existing cholesterol-laden gallstones, the commonest type of gallstones.

Early warning symptoms of gallbladder cancer

There are no early symptoms or signs of gallbladder cancer. However, about half of those individuals who develop gallstones do have attacks of severe abdominal pain during their lifetime, while in the others, the 'silent' gallstones usually remain undetected. Early and curable gallbladder cancers are sometimes found incidentally when cholecystectomy is being done for symptomatic gallstones.

A personal risk list for gallbladder cancer

- *Inherited gallbladder cancer.* Due to an inherited tendency to form cholesterol gallstones as seen among American Indians, Hispanics and some families.
- *Personal health risks.* Gallstones are the most important, though the absolute risk of gallbladder cancer is very low (less than 1% after 20 years). The risk is higher with large gallstones, in the presence of a calcified gallbladder wall, and with gallstones that have remained untreated for three decades or longer.
- *Occupational health risks.* Possibly workers in the automotive, petroleum, rubber and textile industries.
- *Personal lifestyle risks.* Factors which are related to cholesterol

233

gallstone formation, namely multiple pregnancies, obesity, a diet high in calories and low in vegetables, fruit and cereals.

Specific recommendations for primary prevention of gallbladder cancer

* Prevent formation of cholesterol gallstones by attention to overweight and diet (Chapter 6), as well as physical activity (Chapter 9).

Early detection of gallbladder cancer using screening tests

* *Gallbladder ultrasound test.* There is no screening test which will show up a gallbladder cancer. However, ultrasound of the gallbladder will identify cholesterol gallbladder stones with about 95% accuracy. This test causes no discomfort and has no risks or side-effects.
* *Screening recommendations for gallbladder cancer.* As gallstones in Western communities are very common (15% of men and 25% of women over 50 years), and as the lifetime risk for those with gallstones is only about 1%, periodic gallbladder ultrasound of the adult population with no symptoms cannot be recommended on economic grounds alone.
* *Preventive removal of gallbladder (cholecystectomy).* Clearly this cannot be advocated for all who have symptomless gall- stones. Cholecystectomy is performed for those with symptomatic gallstones, who as a bonus receive 'preventive treatment' for gallbladder cancer. Preventive surgery for those known to have cholesterol gallstones is recommended if stones are known to be longstanding (say over 30 years), if larger than 3 cm in size, or if there is calcium seen in the gallbladder wall on ultrasound or x-ray. The number of cholecystectomy operations for gallstones has increased over the years, and gallbladder cancers have decreased, presum- ably as a consequence of reducing the number of men and women whose gallbladders were at risk for that cancer.

KIDNEY CANCER

The kidneys are situated in the back of the abdomen, and their main function is to produce urine (Figure 17). During 1999, about 150,000 men and women will be identified with kidney cancer in the world, and of these about 30,000 will be in the USA, about 5000 in the United Kingdom, and over 1000 in Australia. The outlook for a person who develops kidney cancer is good if it is detected early, whilst the cancer remains within the kidney substance. In about half of those who develop kidney cancer, the tumour remains within the kidney and therefore surgical removal of the kidney will usually cure the individual. Although much can be done even for those in whom the kidney tumour has spread far from the kidney, such as into the lungs, the eventual outlook for these individuals is worse than when the tumour is just within the kidney itself.

Figure 17: The position of the kidneys. The urine produced passes down the ureters, and is collected in the urinary bladder

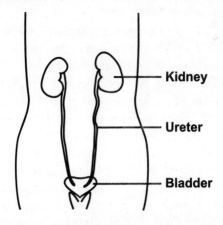

Early warning symptoms and signs of kidney cancer

Unfortunately, in most instances early warning symptoms or signs of this cancer are not present, and in most the tumour remains 'silent' until it is fairly advanced. Pain or aching in the loin, blood in the urine and a swelling in the loin or abdomen are the classic symptoms and signs of kidney cancer, but very often these appear only when there is already an advanced tumour present.

A personal risk list for kidney cancer

- *Inherited kidney cancer.* Very occasionally kidney cancer can occur in families. The mutated gene VHL and in children the WT1 gene appear to be involved in inherited kidney cancer. It can also be one of the cancers which develops as part of the hereditary non-polyposis colorectal cancer syndrome (HNPCC) discussed in Chapters 4 and 14.
- *Occupational health risks.* Workers in the leather, dye, textile, rubber and plastic industries, coke-oven workers, those exposed to cadmium, and possibly those exposed to asbestos, petroleum, tar and pitch products.
- *Personal health risks.* Abuse of phenacetin-containing pain relieving medications (now off the market), long-term use of some diuretics, anti-hypertensives and diet pills. Past history of kidney injury or past history of therapeutic radiation to the kidney region, patients on long-term haemodialysis, or with a past history of large kidney stones.
- *Personal lifestyle risks.* Smoking and being overweight or obese are two important risks for kidney cancer.

Specific recommendations for primary prevention of kidney cancer

- Avoid smoking (Chapter 6).
- Reduce weight with calorie control, low-fat diet (Chapter 5) and regular physical activity (Chapter 9).
- Adhere to all protective measures in all at-risk occupations (Chapter 12).

Early detection of kidney cancer using screening tests

- *Screening tests available.* There are no simple screening tests available at present.
- *Screening recommendations for kidney cancer.* No recommendations can be made at present in the absence of simple and effective screening tests. In the presence of blood in the urine, pain in the loin, or swelling in the loin, an early medical checkup is necessary.

LEUKAEMIAS

Blood consists of fluid and circulating cells of two main types, *red cells* which carry oxygen from the lungs to the tissues and carbon dioxide waste from the tissues to the lungs, and *white cells* which are important in maintaining normal immunity and the defence of the body against illness. Leukaemias are a group of malignant tumours which are cancers of the circulating white blood cells. Leukaemias can be classed as *acute leukaemia,* often with a dramatic beginning and often difficult to treat in the long term, or *chronic leukaemia,* which usually occurs in older age groups, and is usually more amenable to treatment. Leukaemias are further subdivided according to the type of white cell which became cancerous, and of these, *myelocytic leukaemia* and *lymphocytic leukaemia* are the two common cell types.

In this section the primary prevention and possibilities for screening and early detection are considered together for all leukaemias, partly because there is insufficient knowledge of the causes of leukaemias, partly because the causes in different types of leukaemia are similar and overlap, and partly because at present there are no effective screening techniques for early detection of any of the subgroups of leukaemia.

In 1999 about 250,000 individuals will be diagnosed in the world with leukaemia. Of these, 27,000 will be in the USA, about 6000 in the United Kingdom, and about 1000 in Australia.

The outlook for those suffering with an acute leukaemia is worse than for those who have chronic leukaemia. However, great advances have been achieved in treatment during the past two decades, particularly of acute leukaemias, and further advances are expected.

Early warning symptoms and signs of leukaemia

Acute leukaemia symptoms include lassitude, a general feeling of weakness and ill-health, some anaemia and some tendency for abnormal bleeding. One in 10 individuals who are shown to have acute leukaemia are perfectly well, and their leukaemia is identified when a blood test is performed for some unrelated reason. Acute leukaemia is usually identified by a blood test showing an unusually high number of abnormal white cells in the blood. The leukaemia is then confirmed by biopsy of the bone marrow which shows the presence of cancerous white blood cells produced in the bone marrow, from where they enter the circulation.

Chronic leukaemia usually has an insidious onset of symptoms with fatigue, weight loss, night sweats and a slight fever as the commonest symptoms. In many with chronic lymphatic leukaemia, there are often no symptoms of any type for years, and then fatigue and infections develop.

A personal risk list for leukaemia

Unfortunately, little is known about the causes of leukaemia, and in most who develop it, causation cannot be explained.

- *Inherited leukaemia.* This is seen very occasionally, especially with acute leukaemias. The risk is higher in Down's syndrome and some other rare inherited conditions.
- *Occupational health risks.* Workers, such as those in the chemical industry and the shoe trade, in contact with the solvent and chemical agent benzene are at increased risk. (Benzene is also present in unleaded vehicle fuel.) Radiologists, radiographers and uranium miners are at an increased

risk, probably because of exposure to radiation. Electrical and electronic industry workers are also at an increased risk, possibly because of exposure to low frequency electromagnetic fields (EMF). Some pesticides may also cause leukaemias.

- *Personal health risks.* Previous history of radiation either for treatment or excess radiation for diagnostic x-rays. Chemotherapy drugs such as melphalan and chlorambucil, and possibly the antibiotic chloramphenicol and phenylbutazone are risks.
- *Personal lifestyle risks.* Smoking is a possible, but currently unproven risk for leukaemia.

Specific recommendations for primary prevention of leukaemias

- Avoid smoking (Chapter 6).
- Meticulously adhere to workplace prevention practices in relation to exposures such as benzene, radiation and EMF (Chapter 12).

Early detection of leukaemia using screening tests

- *Screening tests available.* No effective screening tests are available at present for the early detection of either acute or chronic leukaemias.
- *Screening recommendations for leukaemia.* Those who experience extreme exposure to occupational hazards which may lead to leukaemia may choose to have medical checks and annual blood examinations after age 40, although the benefit of this has not been established.

LIVER CANCER

The liver is situated under the right diaphragm in the upper part of the abdominal cavity (Figure 18). Primary cancer of the liver, *hepatocellular carcinoma*, is relatively uncommon in developed Western countries such as the USA, where about 10,000 individuals are expected to develop this cancer in 1999, and in Australia where about 250 men and women will develop this cancer during that year. This cancer is much more common in Asia and Africa, very likely because of the high prevalence of hepatitis B, and more recently because of hepatitis C. Globally about 350,000 men and women are expected to develop this cancer each year. Secondary liver cancer (not discussed here) is, however, very common in developed countries, with the primary cancer being in the lung, breast, colon, rectum and other sites.

The outlook in primary liver cancer is often gloomy unless the tumour is identified at a very early stage. A special type of scarring of the liver, *liver cirrhosis*, is a precancerous condition. Cirrhosis can follow liver damage after excessive alcohol consumption or after hepatitis.

Early warning symptoms or signs for liver cancer

The common symptoms in primary liver cancer are abdominal pain or discomfort, weight loss and a general feeling of ill-health, fatigue and loss of appetite. Unfortunately, in many the tumour is symptomless until a fairly advanced stage.

Figure 18: The position of the liver in the abdominal cavity

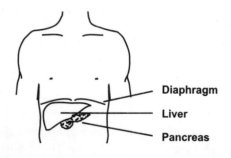

A personal risk list for primary liver cancer

- *Inherited primary liver cancer.* This occurs only occasionally.
- *Personal health risks.* Past hepatitis B infection, past hepatitis C infection, chronic liver disease, liver cirrhosis, and previous steroid use (particularly the androgenic anabolic steroids, and possibly also oral contraceptives). Previous blood transfusion may also be a risk.
- *Personal lifestyle risks.* Excessive alcohol consumption is the most important cause in developed countries, and smoking is a possible additional risk. Staple crops in tropical countries, particularly Africa, when contaminated with a mould which contains a liver toxin, *aflatoxin*, is a risk.

Specific recommendations for prevention of primary liver cancer

- Immunisation against hepatitis is by far the most important preventive measure, especially in those from Asian and African countries where the prevalence of hepatitis is high.
- Limit alcohol consumption (Chapter 7).
- Avoid smoking (Chapter 6).
- Avoid aflatoxin-contaminated food.
- Avoid androgenic anabolic steroids if used for leisure or sporting activities.
- Practise safe sex (Chapter 10).

Early detection of primary liver cancer using screening tests

- *Screening tests available.* No simple effective screening tests are available. A blood test which shows an elevation of *alphafetoprotein* (AFP), has been useful to some extent as a screening method in some high risk countries. Ultrasound examination of the liver is not invasive, it is without risk, and can detect liver cirrhosis or an early primary liver cancer also.

- *Screening recommendations.* There are no screening recommendations in low risk countries such as the USA, Canada, United Kingdom, Australia or New Zealand. In some countries, such as China and Japan, screening with alphafetoprotein (AFP) blood tests has had limited success, especially among those known to have had hepatitis B in the past. In developed Western countries, for those at very high risk for primary liver cancer, such as individuals who have cirrhosis and a previous history of hepatitis B and who are regular alcohol consumers, annual AFP blood tests and annual ultrasound examination of the liver may be reasonable, though these tests have not really been tested as screening measures.

LYMPHOMAS

Lymphomas are primary malignant tumours of the lymph glands. There are two main subgroups of lymphomas, Hodgkin's disease (Hodgkin's lymphoma), and non-Hodgkin's lymphoma.

Malignant lymphomas are relatively common, and worldwide about 350,000 individuals will be diagnosed with these tumours during 1999, of whom there will be about 60,000 in the USA, 7000 in the United Kingdom, and about 2500 in Australia. Non-Hodgkin's lymphomas are more common than is Hodgkin's disease. In the last two decades, much has been achieved with chemotherapy treatment, and this has resulted in long-term remissions and prolongation of life for both Hodgkin's disease and non-Hodgkin's lymphomas.

Early warning symptoms or signs for lymphomas

There are no early warning signs or symptoms. Many who develop lymphomas attend their medical practitioner because of an enlarged lymph gland in the neck, under the armpit or in the groins. A small proportion go to their doctors because they

242

feel generally unwell, have fevers, night sweats and have lost weight.

A personal risk list for lymphomas

Unfortunately the causes of lymphomas are not well understood. Although there is an overlap of known causes between Hodgkin's disease and non-Hodgkin's lymphoma, these will be presented separately. For many individuals who develop lymphomas, causal associations cannot be identified.

Hodgkin's disease

- *Inherited Hodgkin's disease.* Hodgkin's disease can occur in families.
- *Occupational health risks.* Wood workers, rubber workers and chemical workers, particularly those handling tar, and possibly benzene.
- *Personal health risks.* A previous history of tonsil removal, previous use of drugs such as amphetamines and possibly the anti-epilepsy drug, phenytoin. Viral infections such as glandular fever (infectious mononucleosis), the Epstein-Barr virus, or a herpes-like virus. Immune deficiency conditions are also possible causes.

Non-Hodgkin's lymphoma

- *Inherited non-Hodgkin's lymphoma.* This occurs occasionally.
- *Occupational health risks.* Chlorophenols and phenoxyacids, and possibly benzene and asbestos fibre increase the risk. Radiologists, radiographers and uranium miners, probably because of radiation, and electrical and electronic industry workers possibly due to low frequency electromagnetic fields (EMF), are also at an increased risk. Farmers are at an increased risk, probably because of the use of pesticides, herbicides and fertilisers.
- *Personal health risks.* Uncommon viral infections, such as the Epstein-Barr virus, and viruses associated with AIDS. Poor immune state and the use of drugs which depress immunity,

such as those used following kidney transplants in order to avoid rejection of the kidney, and the anti-convulsant drug, phenytoin, carry an increased risk of non-Hodgkin's lymphoma. Radiation treatment is also a hazard.

Specific recommendations for primary prevention of lymphomas

- Meticulous protection from the various occupation-related agents (Chapter 12).
- Practise safe sex (Chapter 10).

Early detection of lymphomas using screening tests

- *Screening tests available.* There are no simple screening tests available.
- *Screening recommendations for lymphomas.* No recommendations can be made at present. Those who feel an enlarged lymph gland in the neck, armpit or groin, are advised to seek early medical attention, which will often result in a biopsy of the lymph gland. If the biopsy is positive for a lymphoma, effective treatment can be commenced early in the course of the cancer, with a high chance of remission.

Mouth and throat cancer

Cancers of the mouth or oral cavity include cancers of the lip, the lining of the mouth, gums, tongue, and the back of the mouth or pharynx (which includes the area of the tonsils and palate), as well as cancers of the throat or larynx. These cancers, whose position in the body is shown in Figure 19, are considered together in this section. Mouth and throat cancers are usually of a similar cell type, squamous cell cancers, and their main causes are similar. Tobacco use and excessive alcohol consumption are important causes in all these cancers.

Humphrey Bogart died of a throat cancer, and he used both tobacco and alcohol.

Figure 19: The anatomy of the mouth, tongue, pharynx and larynx

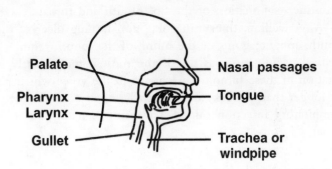

These cancers are not common in developed Western countries, but they are common in the rest of the world, particularly on the Indian subcontinent and to a lesser extent in Asia and some parts of Africa. During 1999 about 500,000 men and women will be diagnosed with these cancers globally, and of these over 40,000 will occur in the USA, almost 4000 in the United Kingdom and over 1000 in Australia. These cancers are usually seen after the age of 50 years.

Precancerous conditions are common for the lip, inside of the mouth and the tongue. They usually reveal themselves as white or grey patches on the surface, as if someone had painted on white or grey paint, which had then dried. These white or grey patches are called *leucoplakia,* and if left unattended, some of these become cancers. On the vocal cords, warts or polyps which are called *papillomas* and which may have a viral origin, were thought to be precancerous in the past. However, it is now known that they only become cancerous if these papillomas are treated by radiation instead of surgical removal.

The outlook for all these cancers is good if they are detected early, before they have spread locally into the deeper tissues, and before they have spread to the local lymph glands.

Early warning symptoms or signs of mouth and throat cancer

Often there are no early warning symptoms or signs. Early tumours are often picked up by dentists or doctors performing a routine examination of the lip, mouth and throat.

Any swelling, thickening or a non-healing ulcer of the lip, mouth, tongue, gums or the lining of the mouth requires early medical examination, as this is the most common early manifestation of these tumours. A change in the voice which persists for longer than a week, and especially when not associated with a respiratory infection can be a warning sign for cancer of the throat.

A personal risk list for cancer of the mouth and throat

- *Inherited mouth and throat cancer.* Inherited causes have not been identified.
- *Occupational health risks.* Exposure to nickel, possibly asbestos and, in the past, mustard gas manufacture, have been associated with cancer of the throat. Outdoor occupations with excessive exposure to sunlight predispose to lip cancer.
- *Personal health risks.* Previous or current patches of leucoplakia on the lip, mouth and tongue, previously removed cancers of the lip, mouth, tongue and throat, and previous vocal cord papillomas treated by radiation predispose to cancer at these sites. Infection with the Epstein-Barr virus, also a cause of glandular fever, predisposes to cancer of the upper pharynx.
- *Personal lifestyle risks.* Tobacco use of any type, including cigarettes, pipes, cigars, tobacco chewing and use of snuff, are most important causes of all these cancers. Excessive alcohol consumption is a further important risk for all these cancers, and the risk becomes very high with the concurrent use of tobacco and alcohol. Tobacco smoke (passive smoking) probably causes some throat cancers also. Mouth cancer

is common in India, especially in the south, where it is related to the chewing of tobacco mixed with dried betel leaf, areca nut and lime to which various other aromatic substances are also added. Mouth cancer is also common in some parts of Asia in which various forms of tobacco and quid are chewed. Regular use of marijuana is linked with cancer at these sites and it occurs in younger age groups. Excessive sunlight is a cause of lip cancer. A diet low in vitamin C, vitamin E, and beta-carotene, which are found in vegetables, fruit and cereals, may also be a contributory cause of these cancers (Chapter 5).

Specific recommendations for primary prevention of mouth and throat cancer

- Avoid smoking and tobacco use in all its forms, and avoid all tobacco smoke (Chapter 6).
- Avoid excessive alcohol consumption (Chapter 7).
- Avoid marijuana smoking.
- Avoid excessive exposure to direct sunlight and use sunscreen on lips when outdoors.
- Eat a diet containing lots of vegetables, fruit and cereals (Chapter 5).
- Retinoids derived from vitamin A or synthetic retinoids taken as supplements are being tested at present in the USA and depending on the final results, may be used in the future for those at high risk of developing these cancers. Recent research suggests that dietary changes, together with the use of synthetic retinoids, have been able to reverse precancerous conditions of the mouth and throat.

Early detection of mouth and throat cancer using screening tests

- *Screening tests available.* Clinical examination of the lips, inside of the mouth, gums and tongue, as well as the front part of the pharynx in the area of the tonsils is a simple test. The back of the tongue, the lower part of the pharynx and the larynx or throat can be examined using special mirrors. Any suspicious swelling, thickening or ulceration can be removed for biopsy.

- *Screening recommendations.* No recommendations need be made for those who are not at higher than average risk for these cancers. It would be reasonable that heavy users of tobacco, heavy consumers of alcohol, habitual users of marijuana, and those with excessive exposure to sunlight as an occupational risk, and other occupational risks mentioned above, have yearly medical checks of the lips, mouth, gums and tongue after the age of 50. Any swelling, thickening, plaque formation or ulceration of the lips, mouth, gums or tongue and any voice change which persists for longer than a week, require early medical examination.

OESOPHAGUS OR GULLET CANCER

The oesophagus or gullet transmits swallowed chewed food from the mouth into the stomach. It is located in the chest cavity, as shown in Figure 20.

In Western countries such as the USA, Canada, United Kingdom, Australia and New Zealand, gullet cancer is relatively

Figure 20: The position of the oesophagus or gullet in the chest cavity

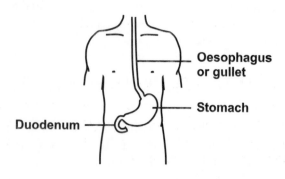

uncommon, and about 12,000 individuals are expected to develop it in the USA in 1999, about 6000 in the United Kingdom and about 700 in Australia. In some parts of China and in parts of Iran and Turkey along the southern coast of the Caspian Sea, gullet cancer is extremely common. Over 300,000 individuals will be diagnosed globally with this cancer during 1999. The outlook if gullet cancer is identified very early is good, but once the cancer has spread through the wall of the gullet, and further, the outlook is much less favourable.

Precancerous conditions are uncommon, the most important being a *Barrett's oesophagus*, named after the English chest surgeon, Sir Norman Barrett, who first emphasised the importance of this condition. In Barrett's oesophagus there is usually a long history of heartburn and reflux of gastric juice into the lower part of the gullet, with a change in the lining cells of the lower gullet predisposing the individual to gullet cancer. Other precancerous conditions are longstanding scarring, inflammation, and narrowing or abnormal pouches present in the gullet.

Early warning symptoms or signs of gullet cancer

Although swallowing difficulty is the most common symptom of gullet cancer, in many individuals the cancer is 'silent' in its early stages. Persistent heartburn, indigestion or regurgitation of food are other symptoms of this cancer, although these symptoms are not specific to gullet cancer, and are in fact usually due to non-cancerous conditions.

A personal risk list for oesophagus cancer

- *Inherited oesophagus cancer.* Inherited causes have not been identified.
- *Personal health risks.* Past history of biopsy-proven Barrett's oesophagus, endoscopy-proven reflux with inflammation of the gullet, many years of marked heartburn, known longstanding previous scarring, narrowing, chronic inflammation or outpouching of the gullet.

- *Personal lifestyle risks.* Excessive alcohol intake and tobacco use are the important risks. The risk is especially high if both tobacco and alcohol are used together. A diet high in smoked, pickled, preserved or cured foods, and low in beta-carotene, vitamin C and vitamin E containing foods (Chapter 5) is also a risk.

Specific recommendations for primary prevention of oesophagus cancer

- Limit alcohol consumption (Chapter 7).
- Avoid tobacco use (Chapter 6).
- Limit consumption of smoked, pickled, heavily salted, cured and preserved foods.
- Eat plenty of vitamin C, vitamin E and beta-carotene containing foods, mainly vegetables, fruit and cereals (Chapter 5).

Early detection of oesophagus cancer using screening tests

- *Screening tests available.* There are no simple screening tests for cancer of the gullet. These cancers are identified by flexible endoscopy and biopsy of any suspicious parts of the gullet lining.
- *Screening recommendations.* There are no specific screening recommendations for those who do not have symptoms, have no special risk factors, and do not have any precancerous conditions. For those who have been identified with Barrett's oesophagus, a flexible endoscopy of the upper gastrointestinal tract involving the gullet and the stomach is recommended annually from the time of diagnosis.

PANCREAS CANCER

The pancreas is an important organ located in the upper part of the abdominal cavity (Figure 21). It manufactures insulin and also several enzymes concerned in the digestion of food. In 1999 about 200,000 individuals will develop this cancer in the world. Of these, there will be about 26,000 in the USA, 7000 in the United Kingdom, and 1500 in Australia. Unfortunately, most of these individuals will die of their cancer, since the outlook for pancreatic cancer is poor. Very often there are no early warning symptoms and signs, and there are no known and recognisable precancerous conditions. Moreover, pancreas cancer is often 'silent' until a late stage, when pain, weight loss, ill-health and jaundice are experienced.

Figure 21: The position of the pancreas in the abdominal cavity

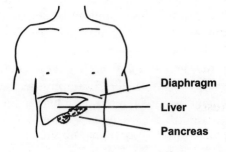

Diaphragm
Liver
Pancreas

A personal risk list for pancreas cancer

- *Inherited primary pancreas cancer.* Occasionally seen in families.
- *Occupational health risks.* Chemical workers, dye workers, nickel, copper, asbestos, uranium and rubber industry workers are at risk. The risk among radiologists and radiographers is elevated (Chapter 12).
- *Personal health risks.* Diabetes and chronic pancreatitis.
- *Personal lifestyle risks.* Smoking is the most important risk for pancreas cancer. Diet is also a factor, particularly a high fat, high meat, and low vegetable and fruit diet. A very high alcohol intake over many years possibly increases the risk.

251

Specific recommendations for primary prevention of pancreas cancer

- Avoid smoking (Chapter 6).
- Eat a low-fat, low meat, high vegetable, high fruit diet (Chapter 5).
- Moderate alcohol consumption (Chapter 7).
- In occupations at risk for pancreas cancer, use recommended safeguards at work (Chapter 12).

Early detection of pancreas cancer using screening tests

- *Screening tests available.* At present there are no simple screening tests available. Ultrasound and computed tomographic scan of the abdomen are useful for diagnosis. These tests are not cost effective for screening.
- *Screening recommendations.* There are no screening recommendations for pancreas cancer. With any persistent abdominal pain, weight loss or jaundice in adults a medical check is necessary, and this may include ultrasound or computed tomographic scanning of the pancreas.

PENIS CANCER

Cancer of the penis is uncommon in developed Western countries, and particularly so when circumcision together with proper penile hygiene is practised. The outlook for cancer of the penis is usually good if identified early. In spite of the usual obviousness of the tumour, it is often neglected by men. Advanced cancers have a much poorer outlook than early cancers. Precancerous conditions include flat or warty swellings of the end of the penis or foreskin. An abnormal narrowing of the foreskin called *phimosis* can also be regarded as a precancerous condition, probably because the normal secretions under the foreskin cannot be cleaned, and they stagnate.

Early warning symptoms or signs of penis cancer

A swelling, thickening, ulceration or persistent 'rash' of the end of the penis or foreskin are the early symptoms and signs of penis cancer, and need medical attention.

A personal risk list for penis cancer

Penis cancer is very uncommon under the age of 50.

- *Inherited penis cancer.* Inherited factors have not been identified.
- *Occupational health risks.* Farmers are at an increased risk, possibly because of carcinogenic chemicals in fertilisers, pesticides and weed killers.
- *Personal health risks.* Previous papilloma or wart, the human papilloma virus (HPV), genital herpes (herpes simplex II), or a narrowed foreskin in an uncircumcised man are all risks for penis cancer.
- *Personal lifestyle risks.* Poor penile hygiene in an uncircumcised man, homosexuality, and possibly smoking are risk factors.

Specific recommendations for primary prevention of penis cancer

- Occupational safeguards for farmers (Chapter 12).
- Penile hygiene both when circumcised and uncircumcised.
- Avoid smoking (Chapter 6).
- If there is foreskin narrowing which makes penile hygiene difficult, circumcision is recommended.
- Practise safe sex to avoid sexually transmitted conditions, particularly human papilloma virus, warts and genital herpes.

Early detection of penis cancer using screening tests

- *Screening tests available.* Regular inspection and daily penile hygiene will detect any swelling, thickening, lumps, ulcers or rashes of the penis, and under these circumstances an early medical checkup is advised.

- *Screening recommendations.* Regular inspection and daily penile hygiene in all adult men.

SARCOMAS

Sarcomas are malignant tumours which originate in the connective tissues of the body, in bone, cartilage, muscle, blood vessels, fibrous tissue or fatty tissue. These malignant tumours are uncommon, and in 1999 about 9000 individuals will be diagnosed in the USA, about 2000 in the UK and over 500 in Australia. They are of two main types, either *soft tissue sarcomas* that originate in muscle (myosarcoma), fibrous tissue (fibrosarcoma), fatty tissue (liposarcoma) or blood vessels (angiosarcoma), or *solid connective tissue sarcomas* that originate from bone (osteosarcoma), or cartilage (chondrosarcoma). Research about the causes of sarcomas is not well advanced, and therefore primary prevention is not well developed. Simple screening tests are not available. Soft tissue sarcomas and sarcomas in solid connective tissues are described together, because their causes, primary prevention and possibilities for screening overlap. There are some precancerous conditions, particularly for bone or cartilage tumours. The condition of *Paget's disease of bone,* and benign cartilage growths which grow into the bone and which are called *enchondromas,* are precancerous conditions. The common cartilage and bone outgrowths (in contrast to enchondromas) are, however, not usually precancerous. A rare inherited condition with benign tumours of the skin, fibrous tissue and of nerve fibres called *von Recklinghausen's disease*, is also a premalignant condition for sarcomas.

Early warning symptoms and signs of sarcomas

Persistent swelling, thickening, or a lump in a bone, cartilage, muscle, fat or fibrous tissue anywhere in the body needs to be regarded as an early symptom or sign of a sarcoma, although in most cases these lumps, swellings and thickenings do not in fact turn out to be sarcomas.

A personal risk list for sarcomas

Although in many cases a cause is not identified, pre-existing bone and cartilage abnormalities, radiation, some viruses and some chemicals are the most important risks.

- *Inherited sarcomas.* Occasionally there is a family history or an inherited premalignant syndrome such as von Recklinghausen's disease.
- *Occupational health risks.* Herbicides, wood preservatives, radiation and defoliants.
- *Personal health risks.* History of Paget's disease of bone, cartilage growths into the bone, von Recklinghausen's disease, radiation, chemotherapy and HIV progressing to AIDS.
- *Metallic surgical implants.* Bullets and shrapnel in the body.
- *Injury.* Local injury is probably not a risk but sometimes calls attention to a sarcoma which is already present but symptomless.
- *Personal lifestyle risks.* Male homosexuality, AIDS (for Kaposi sarcoma), possibly smoking.

Specific recommendations for primary prevention of sarcomas

- Use all necessary protection in the several at-risk occupations (Chapter 12).
- Avoid or minimise exposure to radiation.
- Avoid smoking (Chapter 6).
- Practise safe sex (Kaposi sarcoma, Chapter 10).

Early detection of sarcomas using screening tests

- *Screening tests available.* There are no simple screening tests. Any persistent lump, swelling or thickening in bone, cartilage, muscle, fat or other tissue of the body requires a medical checkup.

- *Screening recommendations for sarcomas.* No specific screening recommendations can be made at present for average risk individuals. Precancerous conditions of Paget's diease, cartilage growths, von Recklinghausen's disease, or a family history of sarcomas, need annual medical checkups. Lumps, swellings or thickening anywhere persisting for longer than one month need a medical checkup.

TESTICULAR CANCER

Cancers of the testicle are not common, although they are increasing in Western societies. More than 7000 men are expected to be diagnosed with this cancer in the USA in 1999, about 1500 in the United Kingdom and about 500 in Australia. These cancers are most common in young men between the ages of 20 and 35 years. There are two common types: *seminomas* make up two-thirds of the group, whilst *teratomas* form the remaining one-third. The outlook for testicular cancer, if detected early, is very good. If it has spread to the lymph glands or elsewhere, the long-term outlook is more serious, although recent advances in treatment have greatly improved the outlook even in more advanced situations. Precancerous conditions for testicular cancers are found in some infertile men who have a testicular biopsy which reveals abnormal or 'dysplastic' cells.

Early warning symptoms and signs of testicular cancer

A swelling, thickening or a lump in the testicle is the important early warning symptom or sign. Testicular pain can occur but is less frequent than a swelling or a thickening.

A personal risk list for testicular cancer

- *Inherited testicular cancer.* Very rarely, testicular cancer runs in families, and is sometimes also seen in non-identical twins.
- *Occupational health risks.* Vietnam veterans may be at an increased risk. This may be due to the use of defoliants and other similar agents, although this connection has not been proven.
- *Personal health risks.* Undescended or maldescended testicle is the most important personal health risk. Congenital abnormalities of the testicle and mumps orchitis (a viral infection of the testicle), are also important risk factors. Previous cancer in the other testicle is a risk. The sons of mothers who used the anti-abortion hormone diethylstilboestrol (DES) during pregnancy are at an increased risk for testicular cancer. This drug was used over a 20-year period until it was discontinued in the early 1960s. It has also been recently suggested, but so far unproven, that synthetic oestrogens in food are a risk for testicular cancer. Testicular injury is probably not a cause of testicular cancer, but it may bring a tumour already present to the notice of that individual.
- *Personal lifestyle risks.* A sedentary lifestyle and wearing tight underpants have been suggested, but so far unproven, risk factors.

Specific recommendations for primary prevention of testicular cancer

- Exercise caution with insecticides, herbicides and defoliants (Chapter 12).
- Lead a physically active life (Chapter 9).

Early detection of testicular cancer using screening tests

- *Screening tests available.* Testicular self-examination is a so far unproven, but simple, and harmless screening test for testicular cancer and can best be done after a warm shower or bath which relaxes the skin of the scrotum. Each testicle can then be examined individually between the thumb and fingers by 'rolling' it with the thumb on top and the fingers behind the testicle. Note any abnormal swelling, thickening or lumps. However, do not mistake the sausage-shaped, slightly curved structure called the *epididymis* for a lump. The epididymis is usually situated behind the testicle and attached to it, but is not an integral part of the egg-shaped testicle. Any unusual swelling or thickening needs an urgent medical examination. The testicle can be further examined by an ultrasound test which may need to be followed by a needle biopsy or perhaps surgical biopsy of the lump.

* *Screening recommendations.* Testicular self-examination once per month commencing at age 20 until age 50. *Most importantly, urgent medical attention is necessary at any time, and at any age, if a lump or a swelling is felt in a testicle.*

THYROID CANCER

The thyroid gland is situated in the lower part of the neck (Figure 22). It produces a hormone, *thyroxine*, which regulates the metabolic rate or the speed with which the various chemical processes take place in the body. During 1999 it is expected that over 15,000 North Americans will be diagnosed with thyroid cancer, about 1000 people in the United Kingdom, and about 400 in Australia. Thyroid cancer is more common in women than in men. Most instances are seen in those between the ages of 25 and 65, with peaks in early adult life and in the over 60s. The outlook for those in the younger age group is usually much better than for those who develop this cancer at an older age. The cancer cells appear to be much more aggressive in their behaviour when thyroid cancer develops in the older age group.

Precancerous conditions are *goitres*, non-tumour enlargements of the thyroid, and benign tumours of the thyroid,

Figure 22: The position of the thyroid gland in the neck

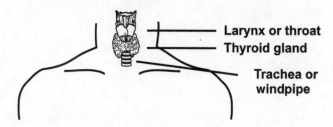

adenomas. Chronic inflammations or immune responses of the thyroid, *immune thyroiditis,* can sometimes lead to the unusual condition of lymphoma of the thyroid gland.

Early warning symptoms and signs of thyroid cancer

Not infrequently, and especially in older age groups, thyroid cancer has no early symptoms or signs. Warning symptoms and signs are a swelling, a thickening or a lump in the region of the thyroid gland.

A personal risk list for thyroid cancer

- *Inherited thyroid cancer.* This occurs occasionally in the younger age groups with one type of thyroid cancer, *familial medullary thyroid cancer.* The mutated gene, *ret,* appears to be involved.
- *Occupational health risks.* Radiologists, radiographers and those involved in uranium mining are at an increased risk due to radiation exposure.
- *Personal health risks.* A previous history of goitre, thyrotoxicosis, thyroiditis or radiation given as treatment for head and neck conditions. Since 1987 over 1000 children have developed thyroid cancer in the Chernobyl region.
- *Personal lifestyle risks.* Possibly excessive alcohol consumption.

Specific recommendations for primary prevention of thyroid cancer

- Protection in any at-risk occupation (Chapter 12).
- Limit alcohol consumption (Chapter 7).

Early detection of thyroid cancer using screening tests

- *Screening tests available.* The appearance of a lump in the neck should prompt a medical checkup including a thorough neck examination. There are no simple screening tests available at present.
- *Screening recommendations.* There are no recommendations in 'average risk' individuals who have no special risk factors. If an inherited tendency for the uncommon medullary thyroid cancer is suspected, a genetic blood test for a *ret* mutation is advised. If positive, this can be followed by the surgical removal of the thyroid at a young age as a preventive method. In those with previous radiation to the neck, yearly medical checks for any abnormal neck lump or thickening of the thyroid is advised.

CANCER OF THE VAGINA AND VULVA

The vulva is the external part of the female genital system, and continues as the vagina, shown in Figure 23.

Cancers of the vagina and vulva are very uncommon malignant tumours. The outlook for early stage cancers of the vulva and vagina is usually good. However, the outlook becomes much less optimistic with advanced cancers. Precancerous conditions include a thickening of the vulva or vagina, which on biopsy reveals dysplasia.

Figure 23: The position of the vagina and vulva

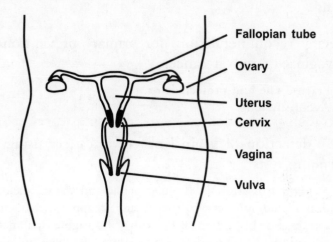

Early warning symptoms and signs of vaginal and vulval cancers

Swelling, thickening, a lump, itching, or abnormal discharge or bleeding are the important symptoms of these two cancers.

A personal risk list for vaginal and vulval cancer

- *Inherited vaginal or vulval cancer.* Inherited factors have not been identified.
- *Personal health risks.* Maternal use of the hormone diethylstilboestrol during pregnancy—this drug was taken off the market in the early 1960s. Previous sexually transmitted diseases, especially human papilloma virus (HPV) and genital herpes (herpes simplex II), are increased risks for these cancers, just as they are for cancer of the cervix. Previous biopsy diagnosis of vulval or vaginal dysplasia (a risk also for cancer of the cervix). Previous radiation treatment given to this area is also a risk.
- *Personal lifestyle risks.* Extensive sexual activity, particularly early in life, with multiple partners and without protection

during sexual intercourse are risks. Smoking is a possible risk.

Specific recommendations for primary prevention of vaginal or vulval cancer

- Practise safe and protected sex.
- Avoid smoking.

Early detection of vaginal or vulval cancer using screening tests

- *Screening tests available.* Regular pelvic and vaginal examination including a cervix smear, and if appropriate, vaginal smears also. Inspection of the vulva and vagina by a medical practitioner. Colposcopy, a procedure in which an optical instrument is used to provide an enlarged view of the vagina and vulva, is a further test which can be performed.
- *Screening recommendations.* For those at high risk, annual medical checkup, vaginal examination, cervix and vaginal smear, starting at age 18. If anything unusual is found, colposcopy and biopsy of any suspicious area may be necessary.

PART IV

A CANCER PREVENTION PROGRAMME

23

A personal cancer prevention programme

And lo! The starry folds reveal
The blazoned truth we hold so dear.
To guard is better than to heal
The shield is nobler than the spear!

Oliver Wendall Holmes (1809–1894)

You are now able to 'tailor' a personal cancer prevention programme, a programme which is pleasant to do, and one which fits in with your specific needs and lifestyle.

Any personal cancer prevention programme also needs to fit into the much broader aim of prevention of all illness and the promotion of good health. A cancer prevention programme should also be enjoyable and easy to achieve in this busy world.

After reading Chapter 3, Who Is At Risk For Cancer?, as well as the subsequent chapters, it is clear that individuals fall into one of two groups—those who have no particular known risk factors, 'average risk', and those who have one or more known personal risk factors, 'higher than average risk'.

Primary prevention recommendations are similar for both 'average risk' and 'higher than average risk' individuals. However, early detection using screening tests can be quite different for the two groups, and frequently depends on the nature of the risk, and on the person involved.

PRIMARY PREVENTION RECOMMENDATIONS FOR EVERYONE

The recommendations in Table 23.1 apply to women and men of all ages whether they are 'average risk' or 'higher than average risk'.

The primary prevention of various cancers can be achieved by decreasing cancer risk through changes in lifestyle (diet, tobacco, alcohol, sun exposure, physical activity, sexual activity, life stresses), changes in the workplace, in the home and in the general environment. The greatest gains can be made in relation to smoking, diet, alcohol, sun exposure and physical activity. These subjects are discussed in great detail in Chapters 5–13 of this book. For certain high risk groups and for certain cancers, some special aspects of these primary prevention recommendations have already been emphasised in the relevant parts of Chapters 14–22. The tables which follow should be looked on as a summary only, and for more detail it would be useful to go back to the relevant chapters.

The message is simple and clear. To lower the chances of developing cancer, eat lots of vegetables, fruits and cereals, eat little fat and meat, be physically active and avoid being overweight, don't smoke, don't drink excessively, avoid too much sun, avoid unsafe sexual practices and protect yourself from any known cancer-producing agents at work, at home or in the neighbourhood. Avoid stressful situations, and practise stress reduction techniques. This can all be done simply and

Table 23.1: Primary prevention recommendations

Diet (Chapter 5)

- Consume plenty of vegetables, fruit, cereals and therefore a diet high in fibre.
- Eat an abundance of foods containing beta-carotene, vitamin C, vitamin E and folic acid (folate).
- For most men, limit energy intake to about 2500 calories per day and for most women, limit energy intake to about 2000 calories per day.
- Keep dietary fat low, not more than 20% of daily calories.
- Keep meat intake low, eat lean meat and skinless chicken.
- Eat low-fat or non-fat dairy products.
- Eat lots of starchy foods, bread, pasta, rice.
- Have a high fish consumption.
- A multivitamin nutritional supplement, which includes vitamin C, vitamin E, and folic acid may be useful for some.

Tobacco (Chapter 6)

- Avoid all tobacco and tobacco smoke.
- Avoid marijuana and snuff.

Alcohol (Chapter 7)

- Drink no more than 3 alcoholic drinks per day if you are a man and no more than 2 if you are a woman.

Too Much Sunshine (Chapter 8)

- Avoid excessive exposure to direct sunlight.
- Cover up when outdoors.
- Use suitable sunscreens.

Physical Activity (Chapter 9)

- For 30 minutes or more, 5 or more days per week enjoy moderate physical activity, such as brisk walking, gentle jogging, swimming, cycling or gymnasium work, which raises your pulse or causes a little sweating.
- Your doctor should first agree that such a physical activity programme is safe for you.

Sexual Activity (Chapter 10)

- Practise 'safe-sex' to avoid sexually transmitted diseases. Some of these can lead to cancer.

Stresses of Life (Chapter 11)

- Avoid stressful life situations whenever possible or practicable.
- Practise daily stress reduction methods which work for you, such as physical activity, enjoyment of hobbies, relaxation, meditation, imagery, yoga, autogenic training.

Table 23.1: Primary prevention recommendations (cont.)

Workplace (Chapter 12)

- Meticulously practise protection from any undue exposure to physical and chemical agents which may cause cancer. If necessary, request information from your employer, union or environmental agency.

Home and Environment (Chapter 13)

- Protect your home and environment from various cancer risks
  - Tobacco smoke—passive smoking
  - Asbestos fibre
  - Radon gas
  - Pesticides
  - Household cleaners, solvents and other chemicals
  - Electromagnetic fields (EMF)

inexpensively, and it can be enjoyable. Simply make all this just a normal part of everyday life. Also, don't forget to laugh and have fun and joy with your family and friends.

RECOMMENDATIONS FOR EARLY DETECTION OF CANCER USING SCREENING TESTS

The recommendations which follow for the detection of various cancers using screening tests, are *not* designed for mass or population screening. They are being recommended for motivated individuals, who after reading this book, in conjunction with their doctor, wish to commence a personal programme for the detection of a precancerous condition, or for the detection of an early cancer.

The first part of this section refers only to those individuals who are at *average risk* and do not have any known cancer risk factors. For those who have known risk factors, that is, they are *higher than average risk*, these recommendations also apply, but have to be modified and enlarged to take account of the particular cancer for which the person may be at risk. In the second part of this subsection, recommendations are made for those who are 'higher than average risk' individuals.

Average risk women and men

This plan includes screening for skin cancers including malignant melanomas (Chapter 18), colon and rectal cancers (Chapter 14), in women, breast cancer (Chapter 15), cervix cancer (Chapter 19), cancer of the uterus and ovaries (Chapter 20), and in men, prostate cancer (Chapter 17), and cancer of the testicle (Chapter 22). In Tables 23.2 and 23.3, men and women are separated, as are different age groups. These tables are designed for quick reference for a particular age group, and are also grouped according to the cancer site. Screening tests cannot usually detect every cancer, nor can they usually exclude the presence of every cancer. Screening tests need to be regarded as something like a net which will trap most tumours or cancers, or which will make one suspect strongly that a precancerous condition or an actual cancer is present. Thus, if a screening test is positive, it usually needs to be followed up by more accurate special investigations which are called *diagnostic tests*. These are tests, such as colonoscopy, upper gastrointestinal tract endoscopy, computed tomography, specialised blood tests and most importantly, biopsy or cytology of a suspicious area in the body, as indicated throughout the book.

Table 23.2: Screening recommendations for average risk men

Cancer site	Age 20–49	Age 50 and over
Skin	• Skin self-examination 6-monthly	• Skin self-examination 6-monthly
Testicle	• Testicular self-examination monthly	• None recommended
Colon Rectum	• None recommended	• Digital rectal examination yearly • Occult blood testing of stool yearly • Flexible sigmoidoscopy at age 50, then 5-yearly
Prostate	• None recommended	• Digital rectal examination yearly • Prostate specific antigen (PSA) blood test yearly

Table 23.3: Screening recommendations for average risk women

Cancer site	Age 20–49		Age 50 and over
Skin	• Skin self-examination 6-monthly		• Skin self-examination 3-monthly
Breast	• 3-monthly breast self-examination (BSE) • 3-yearly medical breast check	• Monthly BSE • Yearly medical breast check • Baseline mammogram age 40, then 2-yearly mammograms	
Cervix Uterus Ovary	• 2-yearly pelvic/vaginal examination and cervix smear (Pap smear) starting at age 20. If 3–4 successive negatives, smears may be done less often, after consultation with your doctor Note: Mainly of value for cervix cancer in these age groups		• Annual pelvic/vaginal examination and cervix smear (Pap smear)
Colon Rectum	• None recommended		• Digital rectal examination yearly • Occult blood testing of stool yearly • Flexible sigmoidoscopy at age 50, then 5-yearly

Higher than average risk women and men

A step-by-step plan for a screening programme follows for those who are deemed to be higher than average risk for cancer.

• Determine that you are a higher than average risk person.

• Use screening tests as described for an average risk person.

- Add a screening programme which is tailored to your individual cancer risk.
- Based on the above, devise a screening plan in consultation with your doctor.

Step 1: Determine that you are a higher than average risk person

An individual may be at a higher than average risk for cancer for one or more reasons, such as an inherited predisposition, or some personal medical conditions, or previous medical or surgical treatments, or some unhealthy life habits, or when that person is subject to workplace, household or neighbourhood cancer risks.

In order to assist with this important task of determining above average risk for some cancers, please use Table 23.4. This table gives a quick guide to the parts of this book which contain the relevant information, so that a sensible assessment of personal cancer risk level can be made. After completing this chapter it is important to verify the assessment with your medical practitioner.

Step 2: Use screening tests described for an average risk person

An individual may be at a higher than average risk for a particular cancer, for example, colorectal cancer, in which case specific screening tests which are probably different from those for the average risk person will be needed for that cancer. However, in all other ways, the screening guidelines for average risk individuals, as set out in Tables 23.2 or 23.3 of this chapter, should be used.

Step 3: Add a screening programme tailored to the higher than average cancer risk

For example, if the higher than average risk is due to a close family member who had colorectal cancer, then large bowel screening consisting of stool occult blood testing and flexible sigmoidoscopy should start at age 40, rather than age 50 as for an individual with average risk for colorectal cancer. Similar

271

Table 23.4: Estimating your cancer risk

Type of risk		Information source in this book	Tick for 'average' cancer risk	Tick for 'higher than average' risk	Pencil in reason for elevated risk and type of cancer, if appropriate
				Check relevant tables and chapters, then:	
Inherited predisposition Family history of cancer		Chapter 3, Tables 3.1 and 3.2 Chapter 4			
Medical conditions		Chapter 3, Table 3.3			
Previous medical or surgical treatment		Chapter 3, Table 3.4			
Life habits	Diet	Chapter 5			
	Smoking	Chapter 6			
	Alcohol	Chapter 7			
	Excessive sun exposure	Chapter 8			
	Physical activity	Chapter 9			
	Sexual activity	Chapter 10			
Workplace cancer risks		Chapter 12			
Household and neighbourhood cancer risks		Chapter 13			

examples can be developed for those at higher than average risk for breast cancer, skin cancer, prostate cancer and others.

Step 4: Develop a plan for cancer screening in consultation with your doctor

Once these steps have been taken, it is best to work out a personal cancer prevention programme with your doctor. Taking this book to the consultation may be helpful.

ILLUSTRATIVE EXAMPLES OF CANCER PREVENTION PROGRAMMES

Average risk person

A 40-year-old woman, who has no known cancer risks and is therefore an 'average risk' person for cancer.

- Primary prevention programme. Use the recommendations for diet, smoking, alcohol, sun exposure, physical activity, sexual activity, life stresses, workplace, home and neighbourhood environment, as summarised in Table 23.1 of this chapter, and described in detail in Chapters 5–13.

- Screening programme. Use screening recommendations for age group 40–49 years, as summarised in Table 23.3 of this chapter, and as described in more detail in the chapters dealing with colorectal cancer (Chapter 14), breast cancer (Chapter 15), malignant melanoma and other skin cancers (Chapter 18), cervix cancer (Chapter 19), and cancer of the uterus and ovaries (Chapter 20).

Higher than average risk person

A 40-year-old man, who is well and has no symptoms, and whose father and brother are known to have colorectal cancer.

- Primary prevention programme. Use the recommendations for primary prevention, regarding diet, smoking, alcohol etc, as summarised in Table 23.1 of this chapter, and described in more detail in Chapters 5–13. Also, pay special attention to dietary changes, smoking cessation, alcohol consumption and physical activity, as described in Chapter 14. You may also wish to discuss with your doctor the possibility of using aspirin as a chemopreventive, as discussed in Chapter 14.

- Screening programme. Colorectal cancer in a father and brother strongly suggests a hereditary predisposition to colorectal cancer. Colonoscopy commencing now, at age 40, and then performed 3-yearly is recommended. Discuss this with your doctor, so that if appropriate, referral can be made to a specialist for colonoscopy and for subsequent surveillance.

Higher than average risk person

A 24-year-old sexually active woman, who is well, and has no symptoms, and who has a past history of genital human papilloma virus (HPV).

- Primary prevention programme. Use the recommendations for primary prevention regarding diet, smoking, alcohol etc, as summarised in Table 23.1 of this chapter, and described in more detail in Chapters 5–13. Also pay special attention to safe sexual practice, avoid smoking, and adhere to the dietary changes, as described in Chapter 19 which deals with cervix cancer.

- Screening programme. History of human papilloma virus (HPV) infection is an important risk for cervix cancer and anal cancer. Annual pelvic/vaginal examination, cervix smear (Pap smear), anal inspection and digital rectal examination is recommended.

A LIFE IN GOOD HEALTH AND HOPEFULLY FREE OF CANCER

> *Trials never end, of course. Unhappiness and misfortune are bound to occur as long as people live, but there is a feeling now, that was not here before, and is not just on the surface of things, but penetrates all the way through: We've won it. It's going to get better now.*
>
> Zen and the Art of Motorcycle Maintenance, *Robert M Pirsig*

Clearly we do not have all the answers to the prevention and early detection of all cancers. However, after reading this book, I hope that you have been persuaded to plan a personal cancer prevention programme. Our current scientific evidence strongly suggests that by using a comprehensive programme of this type, the chances of developing a cancer can be markedly decreased. Using this programme, it is unlikely that a cancer will develop, but if it does it is likely to be identified early, while it is curable. This programme allows one to lead a full, vigorous and enjoyable life.

Glossary

I have tried not to use too many technical or medical terms in this book but inevitably some do need to be used. Readers will also come across these words in the press and in other publications, in TV 'lifestyle' shows, or when talking to doctors. It has been assumed in this book that the reader does not have a medical or biological education, and therefore these alphabetically arranged explanations have been simplified to provide a broad understanding of the terms used.

ADENOCARCINOMA   Cancers which commence in organs and the lining of organs which have glandular structures, such as the stomach, pancreas, colon, rectum, prostate or breast.

ADENOMAS (ADENOMATOUS POLYPS)   Benign tumours which cannot invade the tissues and do not spread elsewhere in the body. They are therefore not malignant and not cancers. When on a stalk an adenoma is called an *adenomatous polyp* and when it grows directly from the lining without a stalk, it is called a *sessile adenoma*. In many parts of the body, benign tumours are precursors of cancer. Removal of precancerous benign tumours, such as adenomatous polyps, is an important means of secondary prevention of cancer at sites such as the colon or rectum.

ANDROGENS Male sex hormones which determine male physical sexual characteristics. *Testosterone* is an important member of this group.

ANTIOXIDANTS These compounds are found in small quantities in vegetables, fruits and some cereals, and are believed to counteract some of the harmful effects of free radicals. Antioxidants include vitamin C, E, beta-carotene, lycopene and the mineral selenium.

ASBESTOS Asbestos is fire and heat resistant and has been used for a long time as a building material and as insulation. If the microscopic fibres of asbestos crumble and are inhaled or ingested, they can lodge in the lungs and possibly in the gastrointestinal system also, and be responsible for lung cancer and mesothelioma—the latter being an uncommon cancer of the lining of the chest—and possibly responsible for some other cancers also.

ASYMPTOMATIC A person who is apparently well and complains of no symptoms.

ATROPHIC GASTRITIS A precancerous condition of the stomach, a result of absent acid in gastric juice, accompanied by a destruction of the lining of stomach glands. Present in pernicious anaemia and some other conditions.

BARIUM ENEMA An x-ray examination of the large bowel, particularly the colon, in which a solution of barium sulphate (opaque to x-rays and showing up white on the x-ray film), is placed into the large bowel through a tube in the rectum, and x-rays are performed. Used as a diagnostic test for inflammatory bowel disease, adenomatous polyps and cancer. Not as accurate as colonoscopy or sigmoidoscopy it is, however, less expensive than these procedures.

BARRETT'S OESOPHAGUS The cells of the lower oesophagus change from an oesophagus (gullet) type of *squamous cell* to a cell of the stomach type or *adeno cell* type. Usually the result of regurgitation of acid from the stomach into the lower gullet. This is a precancerous condition for oesophagus (gullet) cancer.

BASAL CELL CARCINOMA The commonest type of skin cancer. Invades local tissues, and if untreated can cause a lot of disfigurement. This cancer almost never spreads or metastasises to other parts of the body.

BENIGN PROSTATIC ENLARGEMENT (BENIGN PROSTATOMEGALY) An enlargement of the prostate gland, causing difficulties with the urinary stream. This is not a cancer and is not a precancerous condition.

BENIGN TUMOUR This is a tumour, but it is not a cancer, and it never invades surrounding tissues, and never spreads to distant parts of the body. Many, but not all benign tumours, are precancerous conditions, such as adenomatous polyps of the colon or rectum.

BIOPSY A procedure which employs a needle or a surgical cut to remove tissue which is then subjected to microscopic examination. This can make a precise diagnosis that a malignant tumour is present and a *positive biopsy* is rarely incorrect. A *negative biopsy* result usually means that a tumour is not present. In some cases, however, the needle or the knife inadvertently removes non-cancerous tissue adjacent to a cancer, and this is called a *false negative* result, and can occur with small cancers. Almost any tissue in the body can be biopsied.

BREAST LUMPECTOMY A surgical operation in which only the breast lump is removed and the rest of the breast remains. This is a method of breast conservation in some instances of early breast cancer.

BRONCHOSCOPY A flexible optical instrument is passed down the air pipes called the *trachea* and *bronchi* in order to visually diagnose abnormal conditions of the air passages, including lung cancer. During bronchoscopy pieces of tissue can be removed for biopsy. Bronchi can also be washed out, and extruded cells recovered and subjected to microscopic examination in a procedure called *bronchial cytology*, a procedure which can detect lung cancer cells.

CANCER   A condition in which there is an uncontrollable division of abnormal body cells which are capable of spreading locally in the tissue of origin, and also into the more distant parts of the body. There are many different types of cancer in different parts of the human body, and no part of the body is immune from the development of a cancer. The most common type of cancer is called *carcinoma*. Other less common types of cancer are called *leukaemia, lymphoma, melanoma* and *sarcoma*. For a more detailed description of cancer, see Chapter 1, Why and How Cancer Develops.

CARCINOGEN   A physical or chemical substance such as tobacco, asbestos fibre, benzene, tar, food constituents, radiation etc, which can be a cause of cancer.

CARCINOMA   Medical term for the appearance of the cell in the most common type of cancer. Other cell types are called *sarcoma, melanoma, lymphoma* and *leukaemia*.

CARCINOMA-IN-SITU   These are cancer cells which remain at their site of origin, and these cells have not acquired the capacity to invade the local tissues, nor to spread elsewhere in the body. They represent the first stage in the growth of the cancer, and their complete removal usually results in a cure of the condition.

CELLS   These are microscopic 'building blocks' of the body, which together with connective tissues form various tissues and organs. There are many types of cells, such as muscle cells, bone cells, liver cells, kidney cells, cells which line the stomach or bowel, and others. A series of gene mutations in cells, the result of environmental, lifestyle and inherited causes, can result in the development of a cancer cell. Every cell contains a *nucleus*, which in turn contains chromosomes, each a collection of genes, which control every function of the cell.

CERVIX SMEAR (PAP SMEAR)   Cells or samples taken from the cervix which are then examined microscopically for the presence of cervix cancer, or precancerous changes, by a method called *cytology*.

CHEMOPREVENTION   The use of medication, vitamins or

nutritional supplements, such as aspirin, calcium supplements, or supplements of vitamin C, E and others, which may be used in the primary prevention of various cancers.

CHEMOTHERAPY Refers to a method of cancer treatment with *anticancer drugs*. Chemotherapy is not part of a cancer prevention or early detection programme.

CHROMOSOMES These are structures in the nucleus of the cell which contain genes, consisting of DNA (deoxyribonucleic acid), which in turn control a person's physical and biological characteristics.

'COLD TURKEY' The complete and sudden cessation in the use of an addictive substance, such as tobacco or alcohol.

CONGENITAL A condition which is present at birth. This may be inherited, or it can be acquired whilst the foetus lies in the uterus. An example of an acquired congenital condition is a malformation of the newborn caused by a viral illness of the mother during pregnancy.

COLONOSCOPY A procedure in which a long flexible optical instrument is passed through the anus into the rectum and colon. Used as a diagnostic test for the detection of diseases of the large bowel including benign tumours or adenomas, and cancers of the colon or rectum. Figure 7 in Chapter 14 shows a colonoscope in use.

COLPOSCOPY An optical instrument which magnifies the cervix to better examine suspicious areas which can then be biopsied in order to detect precancerous lesions or early cervix cancer. This instrument can also be used to magnify the vagina and vulva for the examination of any suspicious areas there.

COMPUTED AXIAL TOMOGRAPHY (CAT SCAN) A precise but complex radiological examination which takes transverse or cross sectional 'slices' of various parts of the human body to identify abnormal masses, swellings or tumours, including cancer.

CRUCIFEROUS VEGETABLES Called this because the flowers of these vegetables have the shape of a cross. These are members of the *brassica* family and include cabbage, cauliflower, broccoli, brussel sprouts, kohlrabi, swede, turnip and kale. They have been shown to contain anticancer compounds.

CYST   A round or oval structure of variable size containing fluid. Common in the breast and ovary, usually not cancerous, and usually not a precancerous condition.

CYSTOSCOPY   A diagnostic test with an optical instrument introduced into the bladder to detect abnormal conditions of the bladder, including cancer.

CYTOLOGY   Microscopic examination of any discharge or smear containing cells which may prove to be cancer cells, or precancerous cells. The cervix smear or Papanicolaou smear was the first, and the technique is now also used for the detection of many other cancers, including cancers of the lung, liver, pancreas, lymph glands, breast and others.

DIAGNOSIS   The precise and accurate confirmation of the presence and nature of an illness.

DILATATION AND CURETTAGE (D&C)   A surgical procedure performed by a gynaecologist, in which the lining of the uterus is scraped out with a special instrument, and the tissue subjected to microscopic examination. It is a means of diagnosing various conditions of the uterus, including cancer and precancerous conditions.

DNA (DEOXYRIBONUCLEIC ACID)   Every human cell has a controlling centre, called a *nucleus*, which contains very many *genes* made up of DNA, which determine every function of the cell, and therefore of the body. DNA controls cell division also, and if damaged by agents such as smoking, excessive sunshine etc, cell mutations can take place, and these can eventually result in the development of a cancer.

DYSPLASIA (DYSPLASTIC CELL)   An abnormal looking cell, the result of cell damage and mutations caused by lifestyle or environmental agents such as smoking, radiation etc. Dysplastic cells are usually precancerous. With further DNA damage and further mutations, dysplastic cells can eventually develop into cancer cells.

ELECTROMAGNETIC FIELDS (EMF) These are low frequency magnetic fields created by electric and electronic currents, and occur in proximity to items such as electric and electronic equipment, and overhead high frequency cables. Prolonged and excessive exposure may be a cause of some leukaemias, lymphomas and brain tumours.

ENZYME Substances which cause and determine the rate of chemical change and chemical transformation, such as during the digestion of fats, sugars or proteins.

FAMILIAL ADENOMATOUS POLYPOSIS (FAP) An uncommon inherited condition in which hundreds to thousands of small benign tumours, adenomatous polyps of the colon and rectum, develop at a young age. If untreated there is an almost certain progression to colon or rectal cancer. The condition has been shown to be due to the inheritance of an abnormal gene on chromosome 5. This condition is described in detail in Chapters 4 and 14.

FAMILIAL CANCER (FAMILIAL CANCER SYNDROMES) These are uncommon conditions in which several members of a family develop cancer much more frequently than would be expected by chance alone. These cancers are usually in the same part of the body, such as the colon, breast or skin. Familial cancer syndromes are almost always due to inherited gene mutations. Examples of family cancer syndromes are familial adenomatous polyposis (FAP) and hereditary non-polyposis colorectal cancer (HNPCC) and others, described in Chapter 4.

FALSE NEGATIVE SCREENING TEST A screening test result which falsely indicates that a particular cancer (or premalignant condition) is not present, and as a result the cancer is missed at that examination.

FALSE POSITIVE SCREENING TEST A screening test result which falsely indicates that a particular cancer (or premalignant condition) is present. Such a result usually necessitates further special tests, which then can usually *exclude* the presence of that cancer.

FIBRE This is the undigestible part of vegetables, fruits and cereals, passed out in the stool. There are numerous types of fibre. A high consumption of fibre-containing foods appears to have a preventative action in several illnesses, including adult onset diabetes and some cancers, particularly colorectal cancer and colorectal adenomas.

FIRST DEGREE RELATIVE These are close relatives and include a parent, brother, sister or child.

FREE RADICALS These are unstable molecules searching to unite with electrons in order to become stable, thereby damaging normal cells, and especially cell DNA. This process increases the risk of the development of illnesses, including cancer. Antioxidants can be used, and these may counter some of the effects of free radicals.

GENES Genes are contained in chromosomes. Genes determine and control our physical and biological characteristics, including normal cell division. When cells divide, genes are vulnerable to damage by carcinogens and other substances, and this can result in cell mutations which after several mutations may lead to the development of a cancer cell from a normal cell.

GOITRE An enlargement of the thyroid gland in the neck. It is not a tumour. However, a goitre poses a slightly increased risk for thyroid cancer.

HELICOBACTER PYLORI An abnormal bacterial organism present in the stomach, which can produce an inflammation of the stomach, gastritis, as well as gastric and duodenal ulcers. The presence of these bacteria also increases the risk for stomach (gastric) cancer.

HEREDITARY CONDITION A condition or susceptibility to a condition or illness which may or may not be present at birth, and which is due to abnormal genes inherited from a parent.

HEREDITARY NON-POLYPOSIS COLORECTAL CANCER (HNPCC) An uncommon inherited tendency for the development of colon or rectal cancer, and also of some other cancers, particularly cancers of the uterus and ovary in women, and the stomach, pancreas and the urinary system in both sexes. This condition is discussed in detail in Chapters 4 and 14.

HUMAN IMMUNODEFICIENCY VIRUS (HIV)   This virus is transmitted through sexual activity, and particularly unprotected anal sex, and is also transmitted through blood infected with this virus, such as in blood transfusions, and by intravenous drug users sharing needles infected with the virus. It progresses to the usually fatal acquired immunodeficiency syndrome (AIDS), which has been linked with two malignant tumours, namely lymphomas and Kaposi sarcomas.

HUMAN PAPILLOMA VIRUS (HPV)   These viruses are sexually transmitted, and are the most important precursors of cervix cancer. HPV is also one of the precursors of anal cancer and cancer of the penis.

HYPERPLASIA   An abnormal multiplication of cells, a result of cell damage by outside agents such as tobacco, or excessive exposure to sunlight, and it is often the first step in a series of changes which turn a normal cell into a cancer cell.

HYSTERECTOMY   Removal of the uterus. *Subtotal hysterectomy* is removal of the body of the uterus only, leaving the cervix intact, now rarely performed. *Total hysterectomy* means removal of the uterus and cervix. *Radical hysterectomy*, usually performed for a malignant tumour, means removal of the cervix, uterus, upper vagina, the ovaries, and often also the adjacent lymph glands.

IMMUNE SYSTEM   Present throughout the body and consisting of special cells and protein compounds. It forms a most important natural protective mechanism against various illnesses, including cancer. Small numbers of cancer cells can be neutralised or destroyed, especially by the *killer T cells* of the immune system. A sound immune system is essential for maintaining good health and preventing various illnesses, including cancer.

INFLAMMATORY BOWEL DISEASE (IBD)   The two inflammatory conditions of importance are *ulcerative colitis* and *Crohn's disease,* and both of these have an increased risk of colon or rectal cancer in those who have had the condition for several years.

KILLER T CELLS   Circulating white cells, which are part of the cellular immune system of the body. When activated, they can destroy cancer cells.

LAPAROSCOPY   A surgical operation in which an optical instrument is introduced into the abdominal cavity. It is used for the diagnosis or treatment of a variety of conditions, including removal of the gallbladder, division of adhesions, female sterilisation, as well as the diagnosis of cysts and tumours, including cancer, such as cancer of the ovary.

LEUKAEMIA   Cancer of the white blood cells.

LOCALISED CANCER   A cancer which remains only in the primary or original site, such as within the ovary only, within the prostate gland only etc.

LYMPHOMA   Cancer of the cells arising in lymph glands and related tissues.

MALIGNANT TUMOUR   An alternative word for a *cancer* of any type. The cells of a malignant tumour are able to invade adjacent tissues and also to spread throughout the body to distant sites.

MAMMOGRAM   An x-ray of the breast used as a screening test to detect early breast cancer in women without symptoms and without the presence of a lump on physical examination of the breast.

MASTECTOMY   A surgical operation in which the breast or part of the breast is removed. Types of mastectomy include *partial mastectomy*, which is the removal of a part of the breast, *simple mastectomy* or *total mastectomy*, which is removal of the entire breast, and *modified radical mastectomy* which refers to the removal of the entire breast, as well as some chest wall muscles and lymph glands in the armpit. *Radical mastectomy* is the removal of the breast, most chest wall muscles and lymph glands in the armpit, a procedure which is now rarely if ever performed.

MELANOMA (MALIGNANT MELANOMA)   A cancer which arises from the pigment cells of the skin called *melanocytes*.

If untreated it invades the local tissues and spreads or metastasises to distant parts of the body, such as the lymph glands, liver, lung or brain. Usually arises in the skin but can also arise in any part of the body which has pigment cells, such as the mouth, anus or eye.

MENARCHE   Age of onset of menstrual periods.

MENOPAUSE   Age of cessation of menstrual periods, and of a woman's ability to have children.

METASTASIS   A cancer that is distant from the site of the primary cancer, such as a primary lung cancer with a secondary deposit or metastasis in the brain.

METASTATIC CANCER   This is a cancer in which some of the cancer cells have detached themselves from the primary site and lodged in a distant organ, such as a primary rectal cancer with a metastatic growth in the lung, or a lung cancer with a metastatic growth in the brain. Metastatic cancer is sometimes also called *secondary cancer*, and almost always represents an advanced stage of the cancer. The distant lesion itself, or secondary deposit, is called a *metastasis*.

MUTATION   Genes which contain DNA are located on chromosomes of the cell nucleus, and control every function and physical characteristic of every cell. The change in function caused by a mutation is reproduced when the cell divides. While some gene mutations are inherited, many are the result of damage to DNA by agents like tobacco, excessive sunlight, alcohol, radiation and others. Many mutations are not related to cancer, although some mutations are now known to be able to transform a normal cell into a precancerous cell, and then into a cancer cell.

NAEVI   The medical term for skin moles. Some skin moles are precancerous.

NEOPLASM   The biological term for a tumour, and represents a collection of abnormal cells which have escaped from normal control. The process of tumour development is called *neoplasia*. Tumours can be *benign* or *innocent tumours*, and these do not invade tissues and do not spread, or *malignant* tumours, or *cancers* that can invade tissues and spread.

NICOTINE   Substance in tobacco regarded as the addictive element of tobacco use.

NICOTINE PATCH   This can be used as part of a quit smoking programme. It is a skin patch which is applied each day and which releases a decreasing amount of nicotine into the body on successive days of use.

NITRATES   Substances used as preservatives in smoked or cured foods, such as sausages or other meats. When eaten they are converted to *nitrites,* which then may combine with other compounds called *amines* to form *nitrosamines,* which are known to be cancer-producing agents in several parts of the human body.

NITROSAMINES   A family of compounds, some members of which are strong carcinogens in several parts of the body. Some nitrosamines are formed in the body when preservatives which contain nitrates unite with other compounds called amines. Others are consumed, such as nitrosomines found in some foods. Some nitrosamines are inhaled, and pass into the body through the lungs, and these are nitrosamines present in tobacco and tobacco smoke.

NUCLEUS   Is the 'nerve centre' of every cell. The nucleus contains chromosomes, each a collection of many genes consisting of DNA, which control every function of the cell.

OESTROGENS   Important female sex hormones formed during a normal menstrual cycle. Excess oestrogens, when administered medically after menopause, increase the risk of uterine cancer, and increase the risk of breast cancer slightly.

OOPHORECTOMY   An operation in which one or both ovaries are removed.

ORCHIDECTOMY   An operation in which one or both testicles are removed. In cancer treatment, one testicle may be removed because of a cancerous growth in the testicle itself. In the treatment of prostate cancer, removal of both testicles can be used as a form of hormonal treatment to arrest the growth of the cancer.

PAP SMEAR (CERVIX OR PAPANICOLAOU SMEAR) Samples taken from the cervix, with the cells so obtained examined microscopically for the presence of cervix cancer, or of a precancerous condition of the cervix.

PASSIVE SMOKING (ENVIRONMENTAL SMOKE) The inhalation of tobacco smoke, consisting of exhaled smoke of a smoker, and residual or side-stream smoke from cigarettes, cigars or pipes. This type of 'smoking' has been linked to lung and possibly throat cancer.

PERNICIOUS ANAEMIA A condition in which the absence of a specific substance called *intrinsic factor* results in non-production of stomach acid, in the destruction of the acid-producing glands of the stomach, and also in vitamin B12 deficiency. The lining of the stomach degenerates in pernicious anaemia, and this is called *atrophic gastritis*, a precancerous condition for stomach (gastric) cancer.

POLYP Any protruding lump on a stalk arising from the lining of organs such as the colon, rectum, stomach, uterus, cervix or bladder, is called a polyp. This is a generic and descriptive name and does not necessarily mean that it is a cancer or a precancerous condition, as it can also be due to an inflammation. However, a polyp can also refer to a benign tumour, and then it is called an *adenomatous polyp*—this is usually a precancerous condition. A polyp can also be an actual cancer on a stalk.

PRECANCEROUS CONDITION A collection of abnormal mutated cells, a result of cell damage, but not an actual cancer. Can become a cancer over time with further cell damage resulting in further mutations. Precancerous conditions do not invade normal adjacent tissues and do not spread.

PREMALIGNANT CONDITION An alternative term for a *precancerous condition*, described above.

PRIMARY PREVENTION Primary prevention refers to preventing, or at least decreasing the chance of occurrence of a cancer or of its precancerous conditions by avoiding, eliminating, modifying or neutralising the known environmental and lifestyle factors which are the causes of a particular cancer. Examples of primary prevention are quitting smoking for lung cancer, or avoiding cancer-producing diets for colorectal cancer.

PROGESTERONE (OR PROGESTOGENS) Female sex hormones formed in the late part of the menstrual cycle, and also in the latter part of pregnancy. The administration of progestogens with oestrogens in hormone replacement therapy (HRT), appears to decrease the increased risk of cancer of the uterus, a risk which is present if oestrogen alone is given as HRT.

PROSTATECTOMY Surgical removal of the whole or part of the prostate gland.

PROSTATITIS Inflammation of the prostate gland.

RADIATION TREATMENT Refers to one of the ways of treating cancer by radiation, such as x-radiation, radium, or radioactive cobalt treatment. Radiation treatment is not a part of any cancer prevention programme.

RADON GAS The breakdown product of uranium. It can enter a house through the soil or through the water supply, and can be a cause of lung cancer. It can also be the cause of lung cancer among uranium miners.

RECTAL EXAMINATION (DIGITAL RECTAL EXAMINATION) A lubricated gloved finger is introduced through the anus into the rectum by the medical practitioner to detect abnormalities of the lower rectum and prostate, including cancer in these organs.

SARCOMA Cancer of *connective tissues* such as muscles, bones, ligaments, cartilage, fat and fibrous tissue.

SCREENING TEST These are special tests used to detect precancerous conditions and early cancers in apparently well people who do not have any symptoms. These tests must be safe, simple and non-invasive, since we are dealing with individuals who are apparently well. These tests are usually not as accurate as '*diagnostic*' tests and a number of *false positive* and *false negative* results have to be accepted, hence the term *'screening test'*. This means that for most of these tests there will be a number of individuals who test negative for the screening test, and yet in fact they have a cancer, and also that there will be a number of individuals who test positive but subsequent diagnostic tests will not uncover a cancer. *Please note that anyone who has symptoms suggestive of a cancer at a particular site needs to undergo 'diagnostic tests' for cancer rather than 'screening tests'.*

SECOND DEGREE RELATIVE   These are less close blood relatives, and include aunts, uncles, grandparents and grandchildren.

SECONDARY PREVENTION   Refers to the identification and removal of precancerous conditions such as sunspots or adenomatous bowel polyps.

SIGMOIDOSCOPY (FLEXIBLE FIBEROPTIC SIGMOIDOSCOPY)
   A flexible optical instrument which is passed through the anus into the rectum, and then into the lower part of the colon. It is used as a diagnostic test to identify abnormal conditions of these parts of the large bowel, including benign tumours or adenomas, and cancers. The reach of the flexible sigmoidoscope is up to 60 cm or 24 inches, as shown in Figure 6, Chapter 14.

SQUAMOUS CELL CARCINOMA   A cancer arising from the flat squamous type cell found in the skin, gullet (oesophagus), cervix and some other organs. The commonest site is squamous cell carcinoma of the skin.

STAGING OF CANCER   The extent of a particular cancer in the body. Staging of a particular cancer usually relies on assessment during a medical checkup, plus special diagnostic investigations such as scans or biopsy, or the actual removal of the cancer. In almost all cancers, the more advanced the cancer stage, the more gloomy the outlook is for the cancer sufferer. However, in many cancers the complete removal of an early stage cancer means an excellent prospect for a permanent cure, hence we make strong efforts to diagnose and treat a cancer at the earliest possible stage.

SUNSPOT (ACTINIC KERATOSIS, SOLAR KERATOSIS)
Thickened scaly skin usually the consequence of sun damage. It is a precancerous condition of the skin.

SYMPTOMATIC INDIVIDUAL   A person who has complaints, such as shortness of breath, bleeding with bowel motions, abdominal pain etc.

TUMOUR   A collection of abnormal cells which have escaped from normal control when dividing. Tumours are put into two main groups, *benign tumours* such as colorectal adenomatous polyps which remain local, do not invade tissues and do not spread in the body, or *malignant tumours,* or *cancers,* which can invade adjacent tissues and spread throughout the body to distant sites.

Further reading

The reading list below consists of three specialist medical books which have current technical information regarding cancer causes, prevention and early detection of cancer, as well as the diagnosis and treatment of various cancers. They are written for a medical readership. Specific scientific articles are not listed because this book, over and above the author's research and experience of the subject, is based on an analysis of well over 1000 such publications. There are also four other books listed for a general readership, two of which are diet recipe books; one has useful tips on weight control and other lifestyle changes, and one is on food and nutrition facts.

MEDICAL TEXTS

De Vita VT Jr, Hellman S, Rosenberg SA (editors)
Cancer: Principles and Practice of Oncology, 5th edition
Lippincott-Raven, Philadelphia 1997
This book is generally regarded by the medical community as the classic reference book on almost all aspects of cancer.

Kune GA
Causes and Control of Colorectal Cancer: A Model for Cancer Prevention
Kluwer Academic Publishers, Boston, Dordrecht, London 1996
A current account of the causes, prevention and early detection of the commonly seen cancers of the colon and rectum. The book highlights how recent scientific studies have shaped our views on the early detection and prevention not only of large bowel cancer, but also of other cancers.

Peckham M, Pinedo H, Veronesi U (editors)
Oxford Textbook of Oncology
Oxford University Press, Oxford 1995
A comprehensive book on all basic science and clinical aspects of cancer written by over 300 international experts.

FOR A GENERAL READERSHIP

Eggar G
Trim for Life
Allen & Unwin, Sydney 1997
Gives over 200 tips on weight control and other lifestyle changes, such as exercise.

Stafford J
Taste of Life
Penguin, Melbourne 1993

Stanton R
GutBuster Recipes
Allen & Unwin, Sydney 1994
These books by Julie Stafford and Rosemary Stanton are just two of several recipe books available, showing us that healthy food can be made interesting, varied and delicious.

Wahlqvist ML (editor)
Food and Nutrition
Allen & Unwin, Sydney 1997
A reference book of food and nutrition, including the history, evolution, social and cultural aspects of food, as well as food composition, food processing, biology of foods and the relevance of food and nutrition in human disease.

Anticancer organisations

The addresses for further information on various aspects of cancer prevention and early detection of cancer in Australia, New Zealand, the UK, the USA and Canada appear below. Informative, current, and generally free pamphlets and booklets can usually also be obtained from most of these sources. It is best to discuss the information so obtained with your medical practitioner.

AUSTRALIA

The best telephone number for information to the public from Cancer Organisations in all parts of Australia is **13 11 20**

BreastScreen Australia

Aims to help women over the age of 50 to detect breast cancer at an early stage and to find cancers that are too small to feel. For information call 13 20 50

National Breast Cancer Centre
PO Box 572
Kings Cross, NSW, 1340
Tel: (02) 9334 1700
Fax (02) 9326 9329
Web site: www.nbcc.org.au/default.htm

Australian Capital Territory

ACT Cancer Society Inc
159 Marobynong Avenue
Kaleen, ACT, 2617
Tel: (02) 6262 2222
Fax: (02) 6262 2223
Web site: www.cancer.org.au

New South Wales

NSW Cancer Council
153–161 Dowling Street
Woolloomooloo, NSW, 2011
Tel: (02) 9334–1900
Web site: www.nswcc.org.au

PO Box 572
Kings Cross, NSW, 2011

Northern Territory

Cancer Council of the Northern Territory
Unit 3/23 Vanderlin Drive
Casuarina, NT, 0810
Tel: (08) 8927–4888
Fax: (08) 8927–4990

PO Box 42719
Casuarina, NT, 0811

Queensland

Queensland Cancer Fund
553 Gregory Terrace
Fortitude Valley, Qld, 4006
Tel: (07) 3258–2200
Fax: (07) 3257–1306

PO Box 201
Spring Hill, Qld, 4004

South Australia

Anti-Cancer Foundation of South Australia
202 Greenhill Road
Eastwood, SA, 5063
Tel: (08) 8291–4111
Fax: (08) 8291–4122
Web site: www.acf.org.au

PO Box 929
Unley, SA, 5061

Tasmania

Cancer Council of Tasmania
140 Bathurst Street
Hobart, Tas., 7000
Tel: (03) 6233–2030
Fax: (03) 6233–2123

Victoria

Anti-Cancer Council of Victoria
1 Rathdowne Street
Carlton South, Vic., 3053
Tel: (03) 9279–1111
Fax: (03) 9279–1270
Web site: www.accv.org.au

Western Australia

Cancer Foundation of Western Australia (Inc.)
334 Rokeby Road
Subiaco, WA, 6008
Tel: (08) 9381–4515
Fax: (08) 9381–4523
Web site: www.cancerwa.asn.au

NEW ZEALAND

Cancer Society of New Zealand Inc.
2nd Floor Molesworth House
Molesworth Street
Wellington
Tel: 04 473–6431
Fax: 04 499–0849
Web site: www.cancernz.org.nz

UNITED KINGDOM

British Association of Cancer United Patients (BACUP)
3 Bath Place
Rivington Street
London EC2A 3JR
Tel: 0171 613–2121
Fax: 0171 696–9002
Web site: www.cancerbacup.org.uk

USA

National Cancer Institute
Telephone in US & Puerto Rico (Monday to Friday 9 am to
4.30 pm local time)
1–800–4CANCER
Web site: www.nci.nih.gov

American Cancer Society
1599 Clifton Road NE
Atlanta, Georgia 30329–4251
Tel: 800–227–2345
Outside USA call: (404) 320–3333
Web site: www.cancer.org

American Institute for Cancer Research
1759 R Street NW
Washington DC 20069
Tel: 800–843–8114
Outside USA call: (202) 328–7744

The Skin Cancer Foundation
PO Box 561
New York NY 10156
Tel: 800 754–6490 (800-SKIN–490)

National Alliance of Breast Cancer Organizations (NABCO)
9 East 37th Street
10th Floor
New York NY 10016
Tel: 800 719–9154
Web site: www.nabco.org

CANADA

Canadian Cancer Society
Suite 200
10 Alcorn Avenue
Toronto, Ontario M4V 3B1
Tel: (416) 961 7223
Fax: (416) 961 4189
Web site: www.cancer.ca

Acknowledgements

If I have seen further,
it is by standing on the shoulders of giants.

Sir Isaac Newton (1642–1727)

It would not have been possible to write this book without the inspiration and contribution provided by many colleagues, associates and friends. The inspiration to do the research, as well as the shaping of my views about the prevention and early detection of cancer came from many, including the late Dr Denis Burkitt MD FRS, Sir Richard Doll MD FRS Oxford, Dr John H Cummings MD Cambridge, Dr Ernst Wynder MD New York, Dr Sidney J Winawer MD New York, and Dr Bruce Armstrong MB DPhil Sydney. I am also grateful to my clinical and research associates with whom I have collaborated for 20 years in the various aspects of cancer prevention and early detection, and in particular I wish to thank Dr Susan Bannerman MA PhD, Dr Luis Vitetta PhD University of Melbourne, and Ms Lyn Watson MSc La Trobe University.

My particular thanks go to several colleagues who over the years helped to shape my views, and more recently also gave their precious time to read either the entire book or chapters of it, and offered constructive suggestions. For their invaluable help in this way, I wish to thank Sir Richard Doll MD FRS Oxford University (*entire book*), Professor Sir Peter Morris FRS Nuffield Professor of Surgery, Oxford University (*entire book*), Professor Avni Sali MB PhD Swinburne University of Technology (*entire book*), Professor Mark L Wahlqvist MD Monash University (*Diet*), Professor Gabor T Kovacs MD Monash University (*Cancer of the Cervix; Cancer of the Uterus and Ovaries*), Dr Gabriel Zipser MB FRCOG (*Cancer of the Cervix; Cancer of the Uterus and Ovaries*), Dr John P Collins MB FRCS University of Melbourne (*Breast Cancer*), Professor Robin Marks MB FRACP University of Melbourne (*Sun Exposure; Malignant Melanoma and Other Skin Cancers*), Dr James St John MB FRCP University of Melbourne (*Inherited Cancer*), Dr Finlay A Macrae MD University of Melbourne (*Cancer of the Colon and Rectum*), Dr Rodney Syme MB FRACS University of Melbourne (*Cancer of the Prostate*), Professor Richard Fox PhD FRACP University of Melbourne (*Prevention and Early Detection of Less Common Cancers*), and last but by no means least, Professor Richard H Rahe MD University of Nevada (*Stress*).

The background research which was necessary in order to write this book was in part funded by the Slezak Trusts, and for this I am grateful to its Trustees, and in particular its Chairman, the Honourable Walter Jona AM PhD (Hon).

I am grateful for permission to reproduce material from *Scientific American* (September 1996 issue) quoted in the Introduction, Warner Chappel for part of the lyrics of 'Smoke, Smoke, Smoke That Cigarette' (Chapter 6), and for part of the lyrics of 'Mad Dogs and Englishmen' by Sir Nöel Coward (Chapter 8), Macmillan (Picador) for a line from *Give War a Chance* by Patrick J O'Rourke (Chapter 10), Little Brown and Company for Figures 6 and 7 modified from *Gastrointestinal Endoscopy for Surgeons* by R K Pearl (Chapter 14), Carcanet Press for two lines from a poem by Robert Graves (Chapter 15), Spinifex Press for an excerpt from the poem 'Uterus' by Jordie Albiston (Chapter 20), Heinemann for a quote from

The Importance of Living by Lin Yutang (Chapter 21), and The Bodley Head, publisher of *Zen and the Art of Motorcycle Maintenance* by Robert M Pirsig (Chapter 23).

The manuscript and its many drafts was produced by my secretary of many years, Elaine Downard. Even during times of great pressure and demand from me she remained cool and gracious, and I thank her for this. She was helped by Bernard Metcalfe in the final preparation of the manuscript for the publishers. I am also grateful to Ms Janna Stickland, University of Melbourne Department of Surgery, for producing the illustrations.

I have had a most positive and cordial relationship with the publishers Allen & Unwin, and in particular I thank Mr Ian Bowring, Publisher, and Ms Rebecca Kaiser, Senior Editor, for their active support.

It is a special pleasure to acknowledge Dr Peter Greenwald MD, Director, Division of Cancer Prevention, National Cancer Institute, USA, for writing the Foreword. Dr Greenwald is an acknowledged world leader in the field of prevention and early detection of cancer, and having him write the Foreword is a great honour for me.

GABRIEL KUNE MD

Index

In the index the letter 'f' refers to a figure, and the letter 't' refers to a table which appears in the text. For example, 5f refers to the figure on page 5, and 14t refers to the table on page 14.